Renal Failure
Who Cares?

RENAL FAILURE~ WHO CARES?

Edited by
F. M. Parsons
C. S. Ogg

Proceedings of a Symposium held at the University of East
Anglia, England, 6–7 April 1982

MTP PRESS LIMITED·LANCASTER·BOSTON·THE HAGUE
International Medical Publishers

Published in the
United Kingdom and Europe by
MTP Press Limited, Falcon House
Lancaster, England

British Library Cataloguing in Publication Data
Renal failure — who cares?
1. Renal insufficiency, Acute — Congresses
I. Parsons, F. M.   II. Ogg, C. S.
616.6'1406   RC918.R4
ISBN 978-94-011-8079-5   ISBN 978-94-011-8077-1 (eBook)
DOI 10.1007/978-94-011-8077-1

Published in the USA by MTP Press
A division of Kluwer Boston Inc
190 Old Derby Street
Hingham, MA 02043, USA

Library of Congress Cataloging in Publication Data
Main entry under title:
Renal failure — who cares?
Proceedings of a symposium sponsored by Travenol Laboratories Ltd.
Includes bibliographies and index.
1. Renal insufficiency — Treatment — Congresses.
2. Renal insuffiency — Treatment — Great Britain — Congresses.
I. Parsons, Frank M.   II. Ogg, Chisholm S.   III. Travenol Laboratories
Ltd.
[DNLM: 1. Kidney failure, Chronic — Congresses. WJ 342 R3926 1982]
RC918.R4R453   1982   362.1'96614   82-20351

Phototypesetting by Georgia Origination, Liverpool

Contents

SESSION FOUR

Psychological, Social and Ethical Aspects

List of Contributors

PROFESSOR G. D'AMICO
Consultant Physician
Ospedale San Carlo
Borromeo, Milan, Italy

MRS J. AUER
Social Worker
Churchill Hospital
Oxford

MR D. BENOLIEL
Transplant Patient

PROFESSOR R. Y. CALNE
Professor of Surgery
Addenbrooke's Hospital
Cambridge

MR L. CARTER-JONES M.P.
Member, All Party Group
for the disabled
House of Commons
London

DR W. CATTELL
Consultant Physician
St Bartholomews Hospital
London

DR J. W. DOBBIE
Consultant Nephrologist
Glasgow Royal Infirmary
Glasgow

PROFESSOR G. R. DUNSTAN
Professor of Moral and Social Theology
Faculty of Theology
Director of the Centre of Law, Medicine
   and Ethics
King's College
London

DR R. GABRIEL
Renal Physician
St Mary's Hospital
London

DR R. GOKAL
Consultant Nephrologist
Manchester Royal Infirmary
Manchester

PROFESSOR A. C. KENNEDY
Professor of Medicine
Glasgow Royal Infirmary
Glasgow

DR P. LITTLE
Haemodialysis Patient

MISS P. M. LOCK
Research Assistant
King's College Hospital
London

MR P. V. MANCINI
Economic Adviser
Department of Health & Social Security
London

PROFESSOR K. O. NOLPH
Professor of Medicine and Director of
   Nephrology
University of Missouri
Columbia, USA

DR C. S. OGG
Renal Physician
Guy's Hospital
London

PROFESSOR D. G. OREOPOULOS
Professor of Medicine
University of Toronto
Canada

MR R. PAGE
Continuous Ambulatory Peritoneal
   Dialysis Patient

DR F. M. PARSONS
Renal Unit Director
Leeds General Infirmary
Leeds

DR V. PARSONS
Consultant Physician
Dulwich Hospital
London

MR B. PEARMAIN
Chairman
National Federation of Kidney Patients'
   Associations

DR G. PINCHERLE
Senior Medical Officer
Department of Health & Social Security
London

DR P. B. PYNSENT
University of East Anglia
Norwich

PROFESSOR J. S. PRYOR
Consultant Physician
Norfolk and Norwich Hospital
Norwich

DR J. WALLS
Consultant Nephrologist
Leicester General Hospital
Leicester

MR L. S. WILSON
Senior Chief Medical Laboratory Scientific
  Officer
Glasgow Royal Infirmary
Glasgow

MISS E. A. WINDER
Nursing Officer
Guy's Hospital
London

MR R. F. M. WOOD
Reader in Surgery and Honorary
  Consultant Surgeon
The John Radcliffe Hospital
Oxford

DR M. A. ZAKI
Postgraduate Research Student
Glasgow Royal Infirmary
Glasgow

Preface

The last 20 years has seen an enormous increase in our knowledge about the management of patients with terminal renal failure. Despite this, even the most successful dialysis and transplant patients require long term specialist supervision so that renal units will have an incremental work load until the death rate of patients undergoing treatment equals the rate of intake of new patients. Furthermore, innumerable conditions which were once regarded as contraindications to therapy may no longer be seen in this light, so that the number of new patients coming forward for treatment each year is increasing rapidly.

Dialysis and transplantation are expensive forms of treatment, in terms of staff, facilities and consumables, and it is therefore inevitable that there will be problems in providing treatment for all who need it. These will be particularly acute in times of economic crisis. This book contains the proceedings of a conference which was set up to explore the difference between the supply and the demand for treatment in the United Kingdom, to compare the situation with that in other countries, to explore possible solutions and possibly assign responsibility for the shortfall and to examine the practical and moral implications of our failure to treat the treatable.

The multidisciplinary audience consisted largely of people who are directly involved with patient care and who daily come face to face with the consequence of inadequate facilities which are not of their choosing. They and their patients can reasonably ask 'Who Cares?'. They may hope that our legislators and the creators of our wealth may read this book and respond appropriately.

In editing these proceedings, we are bound to acknowledge the help that we have received from many people. Among the most important individuals are Jeanette Robertson-Lomax and Tessa Dorcey of Daniel J. Edelman Ltd who acted as the Conference Organizers and Judy Fagleston who undertook the thankless task of transcribing the discussion. We also acknowledge the helpful collaboration of our publisher. However it was Travenol Laboratories that made the meeting possible.

FMP
CSO

SESSION ONE

A Fact Base: Current Requirements in the United Kingdom
Chairman:
W. Cattell

Chairman's Introduction
W. Cattell

It is my privilege to set the ball rolling on this two-day symposium. While it is entitled Renal Failure, the symposium is about renal replacement for people who would otherwise die of kidney failure. There are few who would disagree that the advent of renal replacement therapy over the last 25 years has been one of the major successes of modern medicine, and there are now many thousands of people who would have died had it not been for the advent of dialysis and/or transplantation. But I think there is no reason for us to be complacent about the situation.

In Stirling some five years ago we had the last major overview of the state of the art in the United Kingdom. At Stirling we were not complacent. It was pointed out there that, whilst therapy was successful, there were many problems. Perhaps the major one that concerned a number of people was the extent to which the provision of renal replacement fell short of what we would desire. However, we were not concerned merely with the extent to which people are given the opportunity to go on living, but also with the quality of treatment provided. At Stirling these problems were well aired. We were fortunate, as indeed we are here, to have a multidisciplinary approach. Not only did we have the doctors – or perhaps despite having the doctors – we had lots of patients, nurses, technicians, social workers and others, all of the team which is so critical for the whole gamut of renal replacement.

Many things have happened since Stirling. A lot of dialysis water has gone under the bridge. We have seen the advent of continuous ambulatory peritoneal dialysis, which, despite the doubts about its ultimate success, has

3

been a major advance. On the other side we have had the *Panorama* programme, which was not good news for transplantation. But there have been many other steps forward, perhaps not as big as we would like. It is quite appropriate that 5 years later we should again take a very careful look at the state of play in the United Kingdom.

Have we advanced since Stirling? Some may say yes, some no. Either way I trust that over the next two days we shall have both a critical view of the situation as of 1982 and useful and positive discussion about ways of improving yet further the quality of life of patients with renal failure and the extent to which we can provide for renal replacement.

The first speaker, Frank Parsons from Leeds, is one of the pioneers of renal replacement in the UK. He had the courage to handle the original dialyser, which was something like the largest ever oil barrel wrapped round with a bit of tubing and half-submerged in a horse trough. He has made a major contribution. He has sat at the table where discussions have gone on. I can think of no one more fitting to start this symposium.

1

Five years since Stirling – a progress review
F. M. Parsons

1.1 INTRODUCTION

At the symposium held in Stirling in 1977, the history of the development of haemodialysis and the early use of intravenous therapy in the management of cholera was presented (Parsons, 1978). Five years ago peritoneal dialysis was used infrequently in the United Kingdom (UK) for the longterm management of end-stage renal failure. The first known use of the peritoneal cavity for medicinal purposes was recorded by Warrick (1744). He removed 36 pints (20.4 l) of ascitic fluid by means of a trocar from a certain Jane Roman, aged 50, in Truro. On investigation he found that the ascitic fluid formed a slight coagulum when mixed with either Bristol water or cohore claret, a Bordeaux wine. Within 6 weeks the ascites had returned 'being ready to break their confines'. After removing a further 20 pints (11.4l) Warrick, following up his previous investigation, injected 10–12 pints (5.7–6.8l) of an equal mixture of Bristol water and claret through the trocar. The patient developed acute syncope. On recovering, the patient bravely agreed to a second injection, the claret 'being in double proportion of the water to render it efficacious'. After draining the fluid from the abdomen the procedure was repeated. Five weeks later Warrick, 'finding everything therefore in a favourable way, her appetite well, her urine in due quantity, her breathing clear, and the extreme parts of their natural size, --- left her in pursuit of that health which she soon acquired, and continued to enjoy'. Perhaps the success of this procedure was due to the development of peritoneal adhesions, a complication that physicians would wish to avoid today.

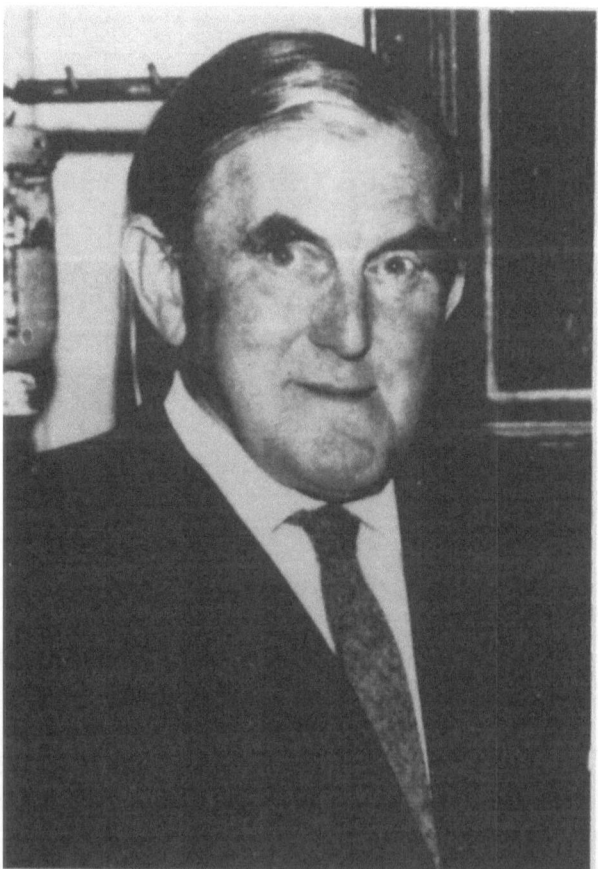

Figure 1.1 Ronnie Reid, urological surgeon, Colchester

The first peritoneal dialysis undertaken in the UK was performed by Reid *et al.* (1946) (Figure 1.1). Later several further successes in the management of acute renal failure were recorded with improvement in technique (Reid, 1948). Unfortunately, further investigations were abandoned (Penfold, J. B., 1980, personal communication) when the dietary regimen for the management of acute renal failure was introduced (Bull *et al.*, 1949).

1.2 UK STATISTICS DURING THE LAST FIVE YEARS

What has happened during the last five years to those patients in the UK who have had the misfortune to develop terminal renal failure? Parkin (1978) attempted to forecast the future in the Stirling conference (Figure 1.2). In 1975 the number of new patients accepted annually in the UK was 14.5 per million of population. Parkin estimated that if this rate of acceptance continued there would be 5000 patients on treatment, by either dialysis or following successful transplantation, in 1980. If, however, the annual increment of new patients continued at the same rate between 1975 and 1980 as in previous years, then by 1980 the UK would have 7000

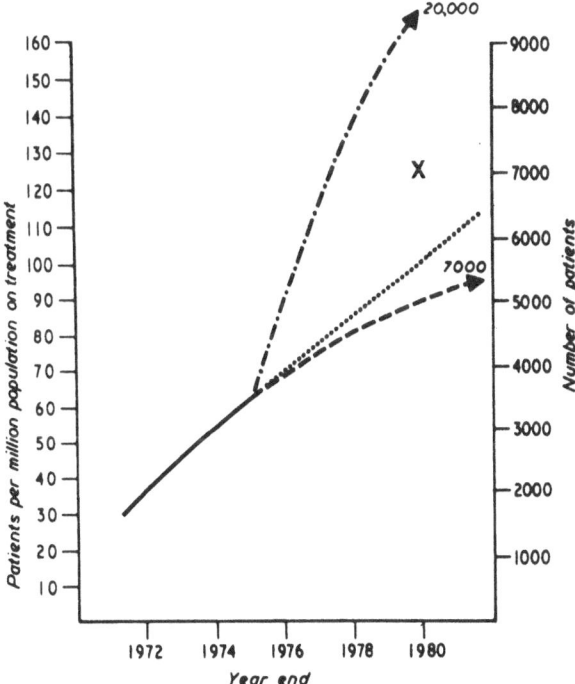

Figure 1.2 Actual and projected numbers of patients treated by dialysis and transplantation in the UK, final equilibrium at 7000 and 20000 respectively (after Parkin, 1978)
---- Projected increase of patients at current intake (14.5 per 10⁶)
.... Projected increase with intake continuing to rise as before
—·— Projected increase with intake of patients = 38 per 10⁶ p a

patients on treatment. This was an accurate forecast, for the EDTA registry recorded that 7146 patients were being treated on 31 December 1980 (as shown by the cross in Figure 1.2, Jacobs *et al.*, 1981). Thus there was no major change in policy between 1975 and 1980. On the other hand, if the UK had increased its annual intake of new patients to 38 per million of population in 1976 and subsequent years (a level which had been achieved in some other countries) Parkin estimated that about 20 000 patients would have been on treatment in 1980 (Figure 1.2). However, the current annual intake of new patients has only reached 24.6 per million of population (Jacobs *et al.*, 1981). No nephrologist finds this acceptable, indeed the UK was bottom of the 16 West European countries mentioned in a recent review

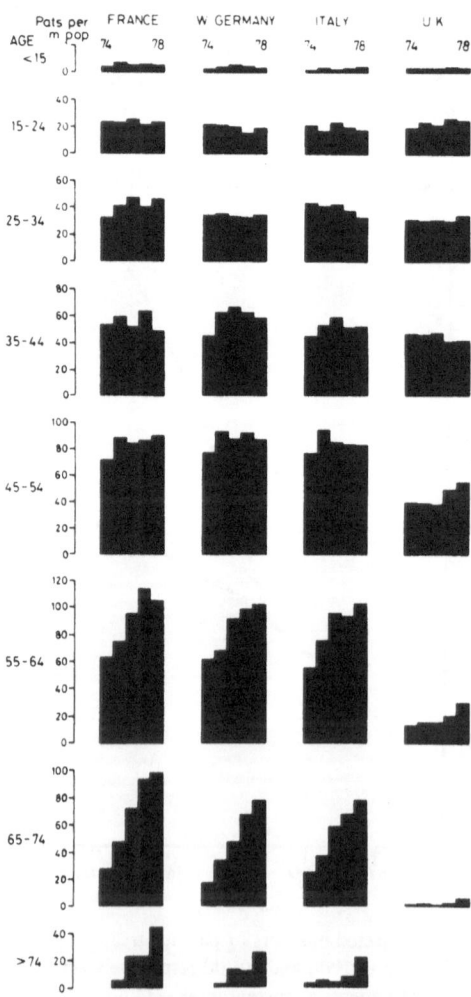

Figure 1.3   The rate of acceptance of new male patients for dialysis in relation to population age structure in four countries, 1974–1978 (Brynger *et al.*, 1980)

(Wing *et al.*, 1981). It is surprising that administrators in our Health Service and politicians have not been active in demanding a better service. They cannot plead ignorance for nephrologists have been very positive in drawing attention to this disgraceful performance in both the medical and the lay press.

1.3 THE MEDICAL PROBLEM

1.3.1 Dialysis requirement

Figure 1.3 records the acceptance of male patients, according to age groups, in France, West Germany, Italy and the UK between 1974 and 1978 (Brynger *et al.*, 1980). The statistics for females are similar except the number of patients is fewer as the incidence of end-stage renal failure is less than that in males. Below the age of 45 the acceptance rate of new patients in the UK is about the same as that recorded for the other three countries. Above the age of 44 there was a dramatic reduction in the acceptance rate in the UK. It must also be noted that the acceptance rates of new patients in France, West Germany and Italy are higher in the decades 45–54, 55–64 and 65–74 than in earlier decades whilst there is also a very profound step-wise increment in the acceptance rates, particularly in the decades 55–64 and 65–74. As there is no evidence to suggest that the incidence of end-stage renal failure is lower in the UK in the over-44 age groups than elsewhere in Europe it is concluded that nephrologists in the UK have not increased acceptance rates for these older age groups. Presumably these older patients are allowed to die. This is a strange ethical problem to occur in a nation that abolished the death penalty, for all types of crime, 25 years ago. There is little difference in the annual cost of maintaining life (and usually a useful, worthwhile life) in patients with end-stage renal failure and of confining in high security prisons those who have offended society. Why has our Parliament allowed this apparent injustice to occur? It is surely against the moral code of all UK citizens.

There could well have been medical reasons for this state of affairs in the UK renal services 12 years ago. The problems created by hepatitis B infection in a renal centre were very real and forced nephrologists in the UK to concentrate on home dialysis and transplantation whilst government seemed to insist on following a policy of financial constraint. Taking data from the EDTA registry reports (Jacobs *et al.*, 1977; Wing *et al.*, 1978: Brunner *et al.*, 1979; Brynger *et al.*, 1980; Jacobs *et al.*, 1981) Figure 1.4 shows that there was no increase in the number of dialysis centres per million of population in the UK between 1976 and 1980 whereas in France the number of dialysis centres per million of population rose from 2.8 in 1976 to 3.5 in 1980. The average number of patients treated by dialysis centres is given in brackets in Figure 1.4. The increase in the average

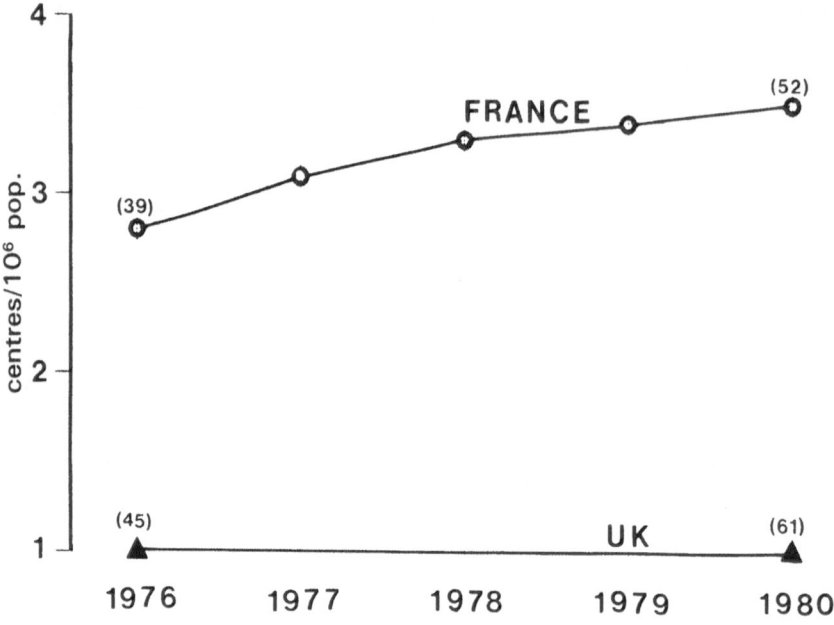

Figure 1.4 Dialysis centres per million of population in the UK and France, 1976–80. The figures in brackets are the average number of patients receiving dialysis per centre.

number of patients treated per dialysis centre rose by 75% in France and 74% in the UK between 1976 and 1980. As this increase was almost identical in the two countries, the rise in intake in the 45 plus age groups in France shown in Figure 1.3 was presumably due to the increase in the number of dialysis centres rather than the number of patients being treated by each centre.

It is emerging from recent, but still somewhat incomplete, statistics that an attempt is being made to correct the low acceptance rate for the 45-and-over age groups in the UK by using continuous ambulatory peritoneal dialysis (CAPD). Although this is a welcome sign it could lead to a major crisis. CAPD is a home-based therapy and so it fits in well within the UK theme, which has concentrated in the past on home haemodialysis. However, all home dialysis programmes require an adequate hospital-based reserve to treat intercurrent disease or social problems. In the case of CAPD, peritonitis is the major complication. If this results in 'drop-outs', and the incidence of 'drop-outs' has been variously quoted, (even as high as 50%, Veitch, 1982), then it is clear that hospital haemodialysis facilities in the UK will be inadequate.

A possible reason for the high number of 'drop-outs' occurring in a CAPD programme is inadequate staffing. Additional nurses and probably additional in-patient hospital beds, are necessary in order to provide a comprehensive CAPD programme in the UK. Too many UK centres are probably attempting to introduce CAPD with inadequate resources. An urgent appraisal by the DHSS is required and if deficiencies are found these must be corrected forthwith. If this is not done then the procedure could well attract, incorrectly, a bad name, besides incurring greater cost.

1.3.2 Transplantation

Transplantation has always played a major part in the management of end-stage renal disease in the UK. The number of patients with a successful transplant exceeds the number on home dialysis (Wing *et al.*, 1983). Unlike the rather abysmal record in dialysis activity recorded above, statistics on renal transplantation in the UK compare very favourably with other countries who provide an integrated programme of dialysis and trans-plantation (Figure 1.5). The DHSS has thrown its full weight behind an excellent publicity programme to expand this form of therapy. A great shame that much of this was dissipated by a current affairs programme on 'brain death' shown on BBC TV (Editorial, 1980). I referred to the pro-gramme as 'journalistic murder', for the subsequent drop in the trans-plantation rate in the UK strained our haemodialysis resources and could well have curtailed the acceptance rate for treating new patients.

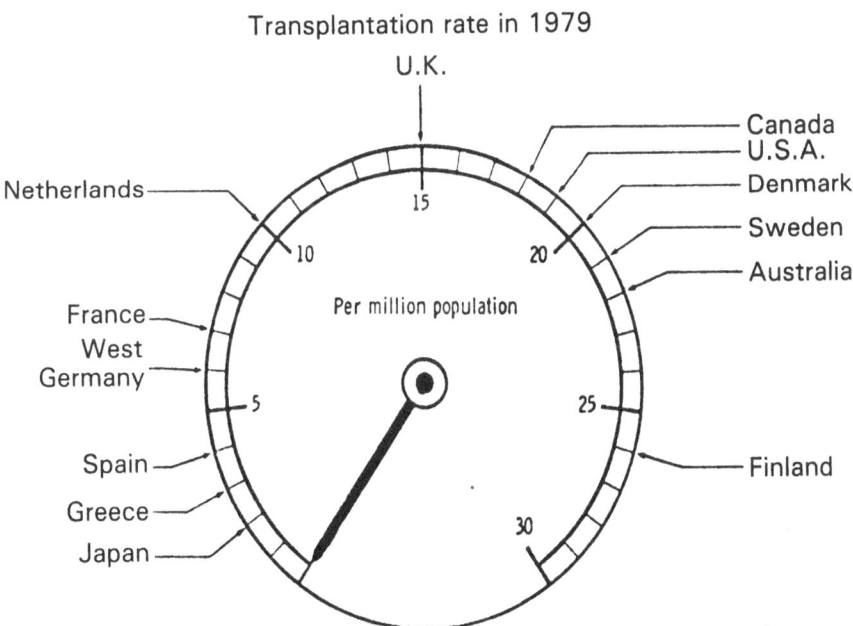

Figure 1.5 Comparison of rates of transplantation in different countries (1979) (Wing *et al.*, 1983)

The number of new transplants undertaken in the UK has remained relatively static over the past 3 years whereas the number of recipients has been increasing, so that by 30 June, 1981 some 2151 patients were waiting for a transplant and even this number was considered an underestimate (Bradley, 1981). A national survey in the UK indicated that many suitable donors are not referred to transplant surgeons when brain death is diagnosed (Jennett, 1981). If more donors became available then dialysis requirements might, seemingly, become less in the UK. However, before this state of affairs arises the intake of new patients per million of population will probably have risen to about 40 per annum. Thus, overall, a further increase in dialysis facilities is inevitable, as any rise in the transplantation rate cannot solve our immediate problems.

Transplantation would play an even more effective role if the rejection rate could be reduced. Professor Calne has updated knowledge of the new immunosuppressive agent, cyclosporin A, in Chapter 10 of this book. The results look most encouraging.

1.4 CLINICAL PROBLEMS

Five years ago many clinical problems were discussed in the Stirling conference. One concerned dialysis encephalopathy. During the past 5 years the incidence of this iatrogenic disease has decreased with the wider use of better pre-treatment of town mains water to remove aluminium. In one of the studies (Ackrill *et al.*, 1980) the use of desferrioxamine as a specific

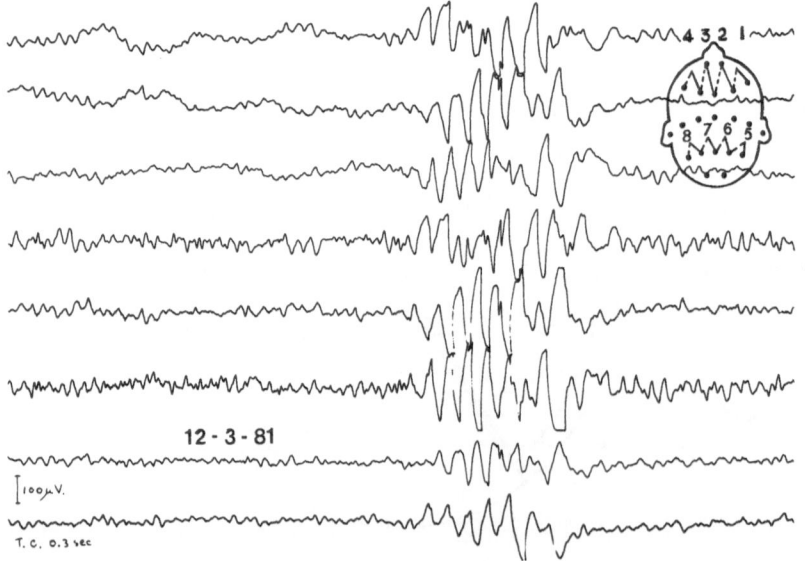

Figure 1.6 EEG of male patient, age 24, who developed dialysis encephalopathy, 12 March, 1981

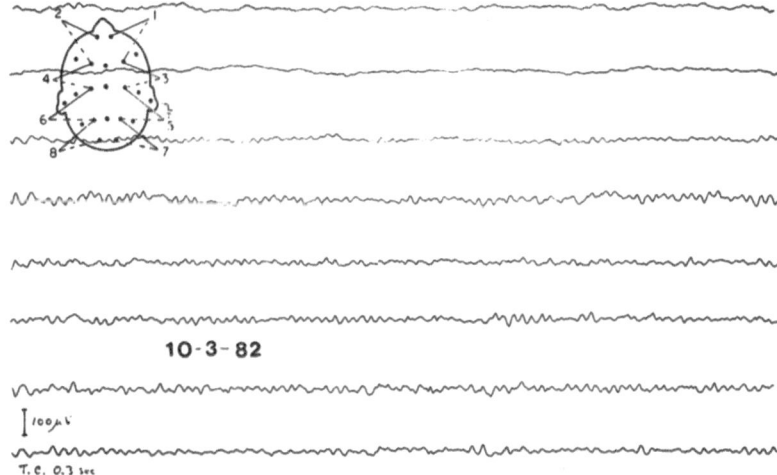

10·3·82

Figure 1.7 EEG of same patient as Figure 1.6, 39 hours post-dialysis, 10 March 1982

therapy for removing aluminium from haemodialysed patients was advocated. One of our patients developed dialysis encephalopathy one year ago and Figure 1.6 shows the classical electroencephalographic (EEG) tracing. Following the administration of desferrioxamine and the commissioning of our recently installed reverse osmosis plant to pre-treat town mains water he lost most of the clinical manifestations of dialysis encephalopathy within 3 months. An EEG taken one year later and 39 hours post-dialysis was almost

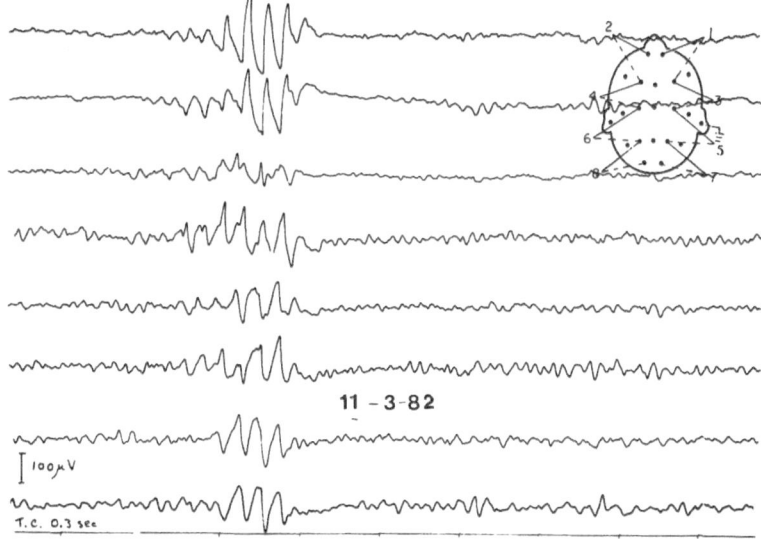

11 – 3·82

Figure 1.8 EEG of same patient as Figures 1.6 and 1.7, 3 hours post-dialysis, 11 March, 1982

normal (Figure 1.7) but a repeat EEG taken the following day but only three hours post-dialysis still showed the classical abnormal tracing (Figure 1.8). Whether this represents permanent damage from aluminium poisoning unmasked by a form of disequilibrium syndrome occurring post-dialysis or inadequate removal of aluminium by one year's treatment with desferrioxamine is not yet clear (Ahmed-Jushuf et al.).

1.5 SUMMARY

The situation currently facing nephrologists in the UK was clearly highlighted by Dr Scribner in 1978. He wrote then, 'who will decide to curtail expenses, and how will the decision be implemented? Significant curtailment is being implemented in the United Kingdom by limiting the dialysis population. The question is, how are they able "to get away with it", and if the real truth were known, could they get away with it?.'

1.6 ACKNOWLEDGEMENTS

Figure 1.1 was kindly supplied by Dr J. B. Penfold, Colchester.

Figure 1.3 is taken from the EDTA registry report X, 1980 and is reproduced by kind permission of the editor of the *Proceedings EDTA* published by Pitman Medical, London.

Figure 1.5 is reproduced by kind permission of the editors of *Replacement of Renal Function by Dialysis,* second edition (in press) and the publishers, Martinus Nijhoff.

References

Ackrill, P., Ralston, A. J., Day, J. P. and Hodge, K. C. (1980). Successful removal of aluminium from patient with dialysis encephalopathy. *Lancet,* 2, 692

Ahmed-Jushuf, I. H., Parsons, F. M. and Exley, K. A. (1982). Desferrioxamine treatment in dialysis encephalopathy. (In preparation)

Bradley, B. A. (1981) Editorial. In Bradley, B. and Moras, D. (eds.) *UK Transplantation Service Review 1981.* pp. 5-8. (UK Transplant Service, S.W. Regional Transfusion Centre, Southmead Rd, Bristol, UK)

Brunner, F. P., Brynger, H., Chantler, C., Donckerwolcke, R. A., Hathway, R. A., Jacobs, C., Selwood, N. H. and Wing, A. J. (1979). Combined report on regular dialysis and transplantation in Europe, IX, 1978. *Proc. Eur. Dial. Transplant Assoc.,* 16, 2

Brynger, H., Brunner, F. P., Chantler, C., Donckerwolcke, R. A., Jacobs, C., Kramer, P., Selwood, N. H. and Wing, A. J. (1980). Combined report on regular dialysis and transplantation in Europe, X, 1979. *Proc. Eur. Dial. Transplant Assoc.,* 17, 2

Bull, G. M., Jockes, A. M. and Lowe, K. G. (1949). Conservative treatment of anuric uraemia. *Lancet,* 2, 229

Editorial (1980). An appalling Panorama. *Br. Med. J.,* 281, 1028

Jacobs, C., Brunner, F. P., Chantler, C., Donckerwolcke, R. A., Gurland, H. J., Hathway, R. A., Selwood, N. H. and Wing, A. J. (1977). Combined report on regular dialysis and transplantation in Europe, VII, 1976. *Proc. Eur. Dial. Transplant Assoc.*, **14**, 3

Jacobs, C., Broyer, M., Brunner, F. P., Brynger, H., Donckerwolcke, R. A., Kramer, P., Selwood, N. H., Wing, A. J. and Blake, P. H. (1981). Combined report on regular dialysis and transplantation in Europe, XI, 1980. *Proc. Eur. Dial. Transplant Assoc.*, **18**, 4

Jennett, B. (1981). Donor supply. In Bradley, B. and Moras, D. (eds.) *UK Transplant Service Review 1981*. pp. 9–24. (UK Transplant Service, S.W. Regional Transfusion Centre, Southmead Rd. Bristol, UK)

Parkin, D. M. (1978). The economics of treating chronic renal failure. In Anderton, J. L., Parsons, F. M. and Jones, D. E. (eds.). *Living with Renal Failure*. pp. 51–65. (Lancaster: MTP Press)

Parsons, F. M. (1978). Introduction. In Anderton, J. L., Parsons, F. M. and Jones, D. E. (eds.). *Living with Renal Failure*. pp. 1–6. (Lancaster: MTP Press)

Reid, R. W. (1948). Transperitoneal dialysis. *Proc. R. Soc. Lond. (Biol.)*, **48**, 413

Reid, R., Penfold, J. B. and Jones, R. N. (1946). Anuria treated by renal decapsulation and peritoneal dialysis. *Lancet*, **2**, 749

Scribner, B. H. (1978). Foreword. In Drukker, W., Parsons, F. M. and Maher, J. F. (eds.). *Replacement of Renal Function by Dialysis*. p. viii. (The Hague, Boston, London: Martinus Nijhoff)

Veitch, A. (1982). *Guardian*, 11 March, p. 2

Warrick, C. (1744). An improvement on the practice of tapping; by which that operation, instead of a relief of symptoms, becomes an absolute cure for an ascites. *Phil. Trans. R. Soc.*, **43**, 12

Wing, A. J., Brunner, F. P., Brynger, H., Chantler, C., Donckerwolcke, R. A., Gurland, H. J., Hathway, R. A., Jacobs, C. and Selwood, N. H. (1978). Combined report on regular dialysis and transplantation in Europe, VIII, 1977. *Proc. Eur. Dial. Transplant Assoc.*, **15**, 3

Wing, A. J., Broyer, M., Brynger, H., Jacobs, C., Selwood, N. H., Brunner, F. P., Donckerwolcke, R. A., Kramer, P. and Blake, P. H. (1981). Treatment of end stage renal failure in the United Kingdom. EDTA Registry analysis. In Bradley, B. and Moras, D. (eds.). *UK Transplant Service Review 1981*. pp. 71–94. (UK Transplant Service, S. W. Regional Transfusion Centre, Southmead Rd, Bristol, UK)

Wing, A. J., Brunner, F. P., Brynger, H., Jacobs, C. and Kramer, P. (1983 in press). Comparative review between dialysis and transplantation. In Drukker, W., Parsons, F. M. and Maher, J. F. (eds.). *Replacement of Renal Function by Dialysis*. (2nd edn). (The Hague, Boston, London: Martinus Nijhoff)

2

Comparison of facilities in the United Kingdom and in Europe for dialysis and transplantation
J. S. Pryor

The overall facilities available for the treatment of end-stage renal failure in most West European countries show great variation.

2.1 HAEMODIALYSIS AND THE NUMBER OF PATIENTS ACCEPTED FOR TREATMENT

The number of patients undergoing treatment by haemodialysis per million of population in the UK on 31 December 1980 (Jacobs *et al.*, 1981) is low

17

Table 2.1 Number of patients undergoing treatment by haemodialysis and transplantation on 31 December, 1980

Country	Population in millions	Number of patients per million of population				
		Hospital dialysis	Home dialysis	Hospital and home dialysis	Functioning transplant	Total
Denmark	5.1	72	19	91	94	185
France	53.3	143	31	174	30	204
Spain	37.1	115	9	124	12	136
Switzerland	6.3	117	32	149	89	238
UK	55.9	23	37	60	56	116

in comparison to the number in Denmark, France, Spain and Switzerland (Table 2.1). This is due to the small number of patients treated by hospital haemodialysis in the UK even though it has the largest number of patients per million of population on home haemodialysis, followed closely by Switzerland and France. Spain has more than twice the total number of patients receiving treatment by haemodialysis than the UK but few are undertaking self-dialysis at home.

The relationship between the total numbers of patients undergoing treatment by dialysis and transplantation in a number of countries and their gross national products (GNP) is shown in Figure 2.1. The UK and France are both close to the regression line and might, from this data, be considered to be placing an appropriate number of patients on treatment according to their national wealth. On the other hand, Spain places more patients on treatment than its GNP would seem able to support whilst Denmark and Switzerland have fewer patients on treatment than might be expected from their wealth. It is noted that the regression line intercepts at

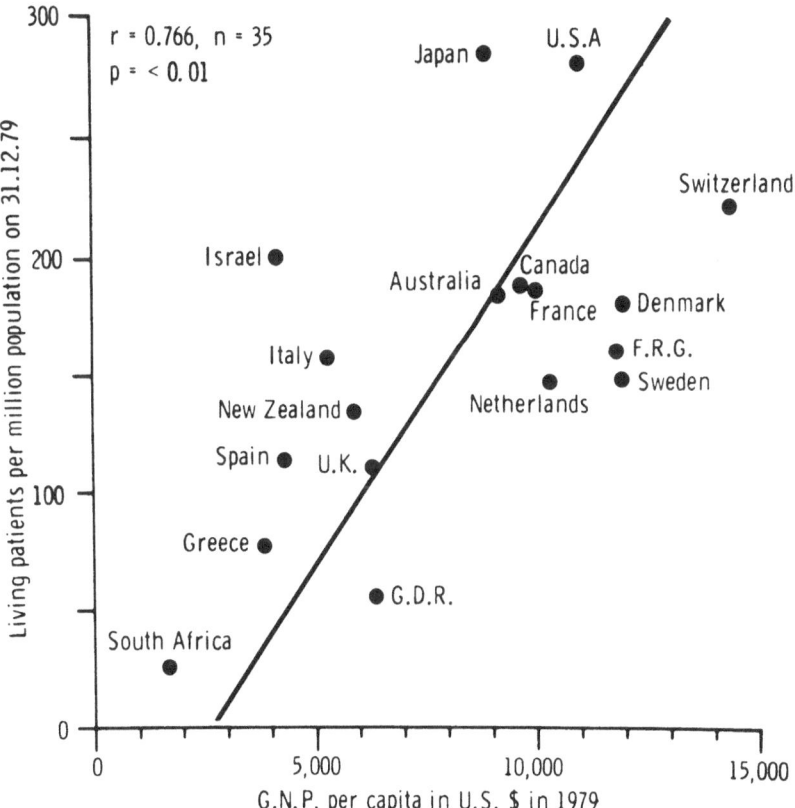

Figure 2.1 Correlation between number of patients alive on treatment for end-stage renal failure and per capita gross national product (GNP)

Table 2.2   Patients starting treatment by dialysis and transplantation during 1980

Country	Patients per million of population
United Kingdom	24.6
Cyprus	56.7
West Germany	44.5
France	42.6
Israel	61.6
Italy	37.0
Norway	38.3
Spain	37.0
Sweden	48.4
Switzerland	48.3

US $2700. Only one quarter of the world's population lives in countries which are more wealthy than this implying that the remainder is unlikely to receive any form of replacement treatment.

Data collected by the European Dialysis and Transplant Association (Table 2.2 derived from Jacobs *et al.*, 1981), indicate that this shortfall is increasing. During 1980, the number of new patients accepted for treatment in the UK was only 24.6 per million population. This figure is approximately half that achieved by Sweden, Switzerland, West Germany and France and substantially less than that achieved even by countries such as Spain and Italy which are sometimes considered to be less developed economically than our own. Data presented elsewhere in this book (Parsons, Chapter 1) suggest that patients aged more than 45 years are the principal victims of this deficiency.

2.1.1   Number of haemodialysis centres

The number of units offering treatment for end-stage renal failure is probably an important factor affecting the ease with which patients can obtain treatment. In the UK the number of centres submitting data to the Registry of the European Dialysis and Transplant Association in 1980 (Jacobs *et al.*, 1981) was 55, each centre treating by hospital and home haemodialysis an average of 61 patients. The figures for France were 179 and 52 respectively, for the Federal Republic of Germany 214 and 49 respectively and for Spain 117 and 39 respectively.

Comparison of the increase in the number of dialysis centres per million of population between 1971 (Brunner *et al.*, 1972) and 1980 (Jacobs *et al.*, 1981) in five European countries are given in Table 2.3. The UK has established only a minimum number of new centres during this 10-year period and this could be one of the main factors leading to its invidious position of currently having about the smallest number of patients on haemodialysis in Western Europe.

Table 2.3 Number of dialysis centres in 1971 and 1980

	No. of dialysis centres per million of population	
	1971	*1980*
Denmark	1.6	2.4
France	1.3	3.5
Spain	0.5	3.8
Switzerland	3.8	4.9
UK	0.8	1.0

2.2 CONTINUOUS AMBULATORY PERITONEAL DIALYSIS

Continuous ambulatory peritoneal dialysis (CAPD) has had a significant impact on the treatment of patients requiring renal substitution therapy. Up to the end of 1980 this treatment was more popular in the UK than in other European countries for over 80% of the UK centres had commenced CAPD programmes. Switzerland was a close second at just over 70% but no more than 50% of centres in other European countries had instituted this form of treatment (Jacobs *et al.*, 1981). The initial popularity of CAPD in the UK was undoubtedly due to the fact that it promised to be relatively cheaper and that it also fitted the basic philosophy of training patients in self-care at home. However, whether this treatment will prove to be successful on a longterm basis and also prove to be more cost-effective has not yet been established. On the other hand, if both these factors turn out favourably then it could allow a welcome expansion of treatment. However, it will probably be necessary to base such treatment on fully established renal centres, which will, eventually, mean a further increase in the number of centres.

Peritonitis is an expensive and disturbing complication for patients receiving this treatment. It occurred in about 50% of patients within the first months of treatment and a third of the patients had up to three episodes of peritonitis. If any complications require hospitalization then the cost of treatment increases accordingly. Finally, the failure to maintain patients on this type of treatment, mainly as a result of peritonitis, is high, possibly 50% at 2 years.

2.3 TRANSPLANTATION

Kidney transplantation is, when successful, the best treatment for patients with end-stage renal failure. If there are no complications it is very cost-effective.

In the UK the number of kidney transplants undertaken in 1980 was 944 (Wing *et al.*, 1981). According to the number of transplants performed per million of population the UK was 7th in the league of Western European countries in 1980 (further comparisons are given in Table 2.1). Unfortunately the number of transplants performed in the UK fell considerably in late 1980 following a controversial television programme. Recovery from this, however, is under way.

One interesting fact about transplantation concerns the significantly better results obtained by transplant centres which performed more than 50 kidney grafts in 1980. There was 75% graft success at 6 months and 66% at 2 years from these units between the years 1978 and 1980 (Jacobs *et al.*, 1981). In centres performing less than 10 grafts per year, graft survival was only 65% at 6 months and 54% at 2 years. This argues for a limited number of transplantation units. It is also accepted that a successful transplantation programme is only achieved when the population is made aware of the need for kidney donors. This will require changes in the law in the UK to facilitate the harvesting of donor kidneys.

Although certain centres are undertaking renal transplantation without an initial period of dialysis, particularly in children, it is necessary to develop a balanced programme of dialysis and transplantation to achieve maximum benefit.

Live donor transplantation gives rise to some difficulties. For example in the Federal Republic of Germany and Switzerland live donor transplantation is not undertaken as it is considered unethical. In the UK 117 live donor transplants were undertaken in 1980, in France 12 and in Italy 17. The numbers of cadaver transplants during 1980 in these countries were 804, 417 and 193 respectively (Jacobs *et al.*, 1981).

2.4 DIABETES

The treatment of renal failure in patients suffering from diabetic nephropathy is a particular problem. Many diabetic patients will develop terminal renal failure and they pose specific problems as a result of their diabetes. The attitude, however, is changing from one of deep pessimism to a more positive and optimistic view. Reasonably successful results are being obtained using dialysis and transplantation procedures.

The use of CAPD for treating diabetics in late-stage renal failure looks interesting. Potentially it offers a means of controlling blood sugar concentrations within a normal range throughout the day. This may help to avert the development of many of the complications of diabetes as well as effectively treating the renal failure.

If CAPD does prove efficacious in treating diabetic renal failure it will mean that even more patients will require treatment.

2.5 CONCLUSIONS

As we view the facilities available to patients who may benefit from the treatments discussed we can but feel rather discouraged by the lack of positive attempts to improve them within our National Health Service.

2.6 ACKNOWLEDGEMENT

Figure 2.1 is taken from the EDTA Registry report, XI, 1981 and is reproduced by kind permission of the editors of the proceedings of the EDTA, published by Pitman Medical, London.

References

Brunner, F. P., Gurland, H. J., Harlen, H., Scharer, K. and Parsons, F. M. (1972). Combined report on regular dialysis in Europe. II. 1971. *Proc. Eur. Dial. Transplant Assoc.*, **9**, 3

Jacobs, C., Broyer, M., Brunner, F. P., Brynger, H., Donckerwolcke, R. A., Kramer, P., Selwood, N. H., Wing, A. J. and Blake, P. H. (1981). Combined report on regular dialysis and transplantation in Europe, XI, 1980. *Proc. Eur. Dial. Transplant Assoc.*, **18**, 2

Wing, A. J., Broyer, M., Brunner, F. P., Brynger, H., Donckerwolcke, R. A., Jacobs, C., Kramer, P., Selwood, N. H. and Blake, P. H. (1981). Treatment of end stage renal failure in the United Kingdom EDTA Registry analysis. In Bradley, B. and Moras, D. (eds.). *UK Transplant Service Review 1981,* pp. 71-94. (UK Transplant Service, S. W. Regional Transfusion Centre, Southmead Rd, Bristol, UK)

3

The costs of treating chronic renal failure
G. Pincherle and P. V. Mancini

3.1 INTRODUCTION

Haemodialysis and kidney transplantation have been available for about 25 years. The development of dialysis has been limited by lack of facilities, trained staff and money, and transplantation has been limited by a lack of cadaver kidneys. However, while this has been clear for many years there have been few attempts to cost these treatments accurately.

Table 3.1 Costs for 1 year's treatment (in pounds sterling)

	1976 study	Study 1976 updated to Nov 1980 prices	1980 treasurers enquiry	Published papers and KCH figures 1980 (see text)	1981 study at one centre at Nov 1980 prices
Hospital dialysis	11 000	19 800	10 900	16 600	9 800
Home dialysis	6000	10 800	5 850	10 900	6450
CAPD	–	–	–	3 300–7 450	5 700
Transplant and 1 year follow up with functioning kidney	3000	5 400	–	5 200	4 700

All costs are for patients established in a particular therapy and exclude extra training costs which may be considerable. Figures have been rounded to the nearest £50. KCH – King's College Hospital.

In an insurance-based health care system some upper estimate of the cost may be obtained from the disbursements made by the insurance carriers. Indeed as far as the carrier is concerned this is the cost. However, beacuse of profit, billing costs and other factors the true cost will be some lesser figure. In the United Kingdom National Health Service (NHS) the estimation of costs is much harder but no less important.

As well as the actual costs of providing the treatment there are many costs falling on parties other than the health services such as local authorities or individuals themselves. These include the costs of social services, travel costs and loss of earnings. While all these and many other items are relevant and important, this paper is only concerned with costs falling to the hospital services of the NHS. It thus presents an incomplete picture and this must be recognized in attempting to draw conclusions from the results.

3.2 BACKGROUND

The Department of Health and Social Security (DHSS) has carried out three studies on cost between 1976 and 1981. These are summarized in Table 3.1. In 1976 we carried out a study (unpublished) in a London teaching hospital, as shown in Table 3.1. The figures obtained exclude capital costs except those of the machines and home conversions, as do all these studies. The figures are subject to many reservations. To facilitate comparisons they are also shown updated to November 1980 prices on the basis of the Price Index for NHS expenditure.

Early in 1980 it became clear that many units had doubts about these estimates which were thought to be too high. Also it was known that dialysers had not increased in price as fast as the Price Index and indeed in some cases, due to bulk purchase contracts, were actually cheaper. The DHSS therefore wrote to the treasurers of all Areas having a dialysis unit for any readily available estimates of their costs. While most Areas sent us some estimates only nine were in a form making them directly comparable. The mean of these nine is quoted in Table 3.1. However, there was a wide range of estimates: £7200–14 500 for hospital dialysis and £2500–8000 for home dialysis.

One of the treasurers referred to above gave an estimate of the costs of continuous ambulatory peritoneal dialysis (CAPD); another estimate, more than twice as high, was published (Gokal et al., 1980). The two estimates showed major differences in accounting practice and staff cost attribution.

A paper from King's College Hospital (Golding and Tosey, 1980) estimated the annual cost of a transplant as £3550. However, this did not include the costs of procuring the kidney or some of the follow up costs and adding these would give a best guess of about £4500. A personal report from this unit gives their 1980–81 costs as £15 500 for a year on hospital dialysis, £10 900 for a year on home dialysis and £5200 for a transplant including one year's follow up but no hospital readmission. This also excludes some of the costs of kidney procurement.

Because of these major differences in 1981 the DHSS set up an in depth study of the costs of three large units which is described in detail in the rest of this paper. Owing to the complexity of the work, provisional results from only one of the units are presently available. These are shown in the last column of Table 3.1. Although these figures are only provisional they support the view that the updated costs based on the 1976 study were indeed too high.

3.3 METHODS USED TO ASSESS COSTS

Between March and September 1981 fieldwork was undertaken at three renal units to extract data on resource use from records of patients with chronic renal failure. The records related to the period 1 April 1978 to 31 December 1980 (33 months). Only one of our hospitals had provided appropriate cost figures for the DHSS' 1980 enquiry.

Hospital A is a large London teaching hospital of over 800 beds, with a nephrology and transplant department and a separate dialysis unit also housing an out-patients department. Tissue typing is undertaken in the main hospital.

Hospital B is a 400 bedded-acute teaching hospital in the midlands with a dialysis unit and adjacent nephrology ward. Tissue typing is done at a nearby teaching hospital which also provides some of the medical staff. Only the data from this hospital have been analysed so far and all the results presented refer solely to this unit.

Hospital C is in the north of England and is on two sites, providing a dialysis and transplant service. The component hospitals are 600 and 800 bedded teaching hospitals. One has nephrology beds in a general ward, for dialysis, pre-dialysis, general nephrology, and transplant in-patients, together with a dialysis training ward. The other site has a nephrology ward and a ward devoted to longterm hospital dialysis for day and night attenders. Tissue typing is done at another location.

For each patient in the sample a diary of treatment events was derived from patient records, and then a 'price-tag' (separately estimated) was attached to each common event, such as an in-patient day or a shunt operation: the total cost of treatment for each patient is the sum of those costed events over the period specified (1 April 1978–31 December 1980). Patients were followed-up from date of entry to the study, to death or to 31 December 1980. The maximum possible period in the study was therefore 33 months.

The costing approach adopted was a 'bottom-up' one, building up the cost of a case from the individual components. This was a retrospective study drawing upon patient records and costing systems not specifically designed for derivation of individual case costs. However, as far as possible, the 'price-tag' or unit costs used were based on unit costs calculated by the finance department for management purposes and usually included in the cost statements. Of course, several adjustments had to be made to the unit costs and in some cases, e.g. dialysis training sessions, unit costs had to be estimated by reference to allocation of staff time, following discussion with unit staff. The events which were identified and recorded are listed in the Appendix.

3.3.1 The samples of patients

All patients whose initial therapy in the renal units for end-stage renal failure (renal replacement therapy) occurred between 1 April 1978 and 31 March 1979 were eligible for the study. Patients whose management had been transferred from other hospitals were excluded, as they were already receiving renal replacement therapy. It had been the intention to study 20–25 patients in each unit. The sample chosen (drawn from the intake during April 1978–March 1979 minus those excluded as explained) is made up of 24 patients from each unit. The sample proportion of the eligible population of chronic renal patients in the units varies from 100% to 40%. Further details of methodology are available, on request, from the authors.

3.4 RESULTS

Only results from hospital B have been analysed so far, so all the following figures relate to this one hospital. Table 3.2 shows how the sample is made up. The mean ages of the patients were very similar to those of the total eligible population. The age range was 21–66 years.

Table 3.2 Composition of sample (patients from hospital B)

	Male	Female	Total	% of eligible patients
Dialysis only no.	7	3	10	59
Mean age	53	47	51	
Transplant no.	9	5	14	47
Mean age	40	41	41	
Total no.	16	8	24	51
Mean age	46	43	43	

3.4.1 Dialysis

The total cost (Table 3.3) of one session of haemodialysis is estimated at November 1981 prices at £73.61 for the training period, £67.95 for routine hospital dialysis and £45.12 for home dialysis. For CAPD the costs are

£60.64 per day during training to which must be added the cost of accommodation in the unit of £46.25 a day and an allowance for drugs, investigations and the initial catheter implantation of £11.30 per day. For routine
CAPD the basic cost of £17.15 a day needs to be increased by an average of
£9.80 per day to cover average in-patient stay, out-patient attendances,
drugs, investigations and operative procedures. The latter figure is however
based on the experiences of only three CAPD patients. For haemodialysis
the average increase to cover equivalent items is £10.75 per session. This
means that the average cost of a week's treatment (three haemodialysis
sessions or 7 days CAPD) is £236 for hospital haemodialysis, £167 for home
haemodialysis and £187 for routine CAPD. It must also be remembered that
there is a cost of about £3286 for three months training for home dialysis;
the cost of training for CAPD including in-patient stay and other on-costs
for three weeks is £2480.

Table 3.3   Cost of dialysis (in pounds sterling)

	Haemodialysis/Session			CAPD/day	
	Hospital training	Hospital routine	Home	Training	Routine
Medical	0.20	0.20	0	0.20	0
Nursing	17.04	11.36	4.93	29.77	0.10
AKAs	4.94	4.94	1.22	–	–
Technicians	2.59	2.59	2.65	–	–
General services	13.96	13.96	–	13.96	–
Consumables	27.86	27.86	27.86	16.60	16.60
Equipment	7.02	7.02	7.02	0.11	0.11
Admin and clerical	–	–	0.45	–	0.34
Home conversions	–	–	0.99	–	–
Total	73.61	67.95	45.12	60.64	17.15

The breakdown of the costs of these modes of treatment is shown in Table
3.3. It will be noted that the major item is consumables. The very high cost
of nursing staff during the training period, particularly for CAPD, is also
important. Also noteworthy is the high cost of general services for patients
treated in hospital.

3.4.2 Transplants

The total cost of a successful cadaver transplant operation is estimated at
£3670. This includes the whole of the in-patient stay of 24 days on average.
Thereafter 'maintenance' costs average £1410 per year. It is probable that
these decrease in subsequent years but the small number of patients and the
relatively short follow-up period do not allow this to be determined.

For unsuccessful transplants the picture is very different, the average cost of the in-patient stay for the operation (29 days) was £4700. Of the five patients studied, in two the grafts failed during this period; a third failed 16 days after discharge – at negligible out-patient cost. However, the other two patients had 195 and 33 in-patient days and 112 and 10 out-patient days respectively from discharge to kidney failure. The costs, following the operative stay, for the patient with the most chequered progress totalled £10850 over a period of 307 days. These five patients were off routine dialysis for an average of 101 days at a cost of £7215 per patient. If the most expensive patient is omitted we find that on average 45 days have been purchased at a cost of £5215.

3.5 DISCUSSION

Much of the data is imperfect and provisional and the patient samples are small in each category so that any conclusions drawn must be treated with great reservations: when the results from the other two units are available it may be possible to be more confident. Nevertheless the figures are of interest not least because they suggest that some common beliefs may be myths.

Table 3.4 shows the 'one year costs' of different forms of treatment. Hospital haemodialysis is, as expected, the most expensive. However, once allowance for complications has been made, CAPD appears to be some 10% more expensive than home haemodialysis. As the data on complications relate to only three patients at a time when the unit had only limited experience of CAPD this may be an unfair comparison and further work is being planned to examine this in more detail. A successful transplant remains the cheapest form of treatment as well as the best from the patient's point of view, however this must be balanced against the costs and hazards of unsuccessful transplants.

Table 3.4 Annual costs (in pounds sterling)

Treatment	First year	Subsequent years
Routine hospital haemodialysis	12 300	12 300
Home haemodialysis (including 3 months training in first year)	9 800	8 700
CAPD (including 3 weeks training in first year)	11 700	9 800
Successful transplant	5 100	1 400
Unsuccessful transplant 101 days of working graft followed by 264 days of home dialysis	13 500	–

The cost for 1 year for 12 patients established on home dialysis will be £117 700. If these patients were to have a transplant on the first day of the year and then had the same experience as the 12 transplant cases analysed here, returning to home dialysis after failure of the grafted kidney, the cost would be £103 300. The financial saving, though considerably reduced, is still present. In subsequent years it would be much greater. Early graft failure produces misery for the patient and high financial cost. Anything which can be done to reduce the failure rate of grafts will thus be doubly welcome.

3.6 ACKNOWLEDGEMENTS

We are most grateful to Mr Mark Davis for help in analysing the basic data and to Mrs Christina Hatchman who typed and retyped our illegible scrawls.

3.6.1 Note

The contents of this paper represent the authors' views alone and in no way commit the Department of Health and Social Security.

3.7 APPENDIX

The 'events' which were identified and recorded were as follows.

Home haemodialysis	– initial operation for shunt/fistula
	– training in hospital
	– routine home dialysis
	– hospital treatment (in-patient/out-patient) for complications, check-ups and renewal of shunt/fistula
Hospital haemodialysis	– the events are similar except that routine hospital dialysis replaces routine home dialysis
CAPD	– initial operation for catheter insertion
	– training period in hospital
	– routine home CAPD
	– hospital treatment for complications, check-ups and catheter renewal
Transplants	– pre-operative stay/assessment
	– organ procurement: live donor/cadaver
	– operation

- post-operative care in transplant unit (and rarely, ICU)
- recovery in ward
- hospital treatment for rejection episodes nephrectomy, check-ups
- post-transplant dialysis, if necessary

It is important to note that patients' records are not always complete – for example records of catheter insertions are not always available: in this case one has to assume that a peritoneal dialysis patient has undergone such an operation:- a similar assumption has to be made about the pre-CAPD-training phase of high-volume continuous IPD, which is not necessarily explicitly recorded.

References

Gokal, R., McHugh, M., Freyer, R., Ward, M. K. and Kerr, D. N. S. (1980). Continuous Ambulatory Peritoneal Dialysis: one year's experience in a UK dialysis unit. *Br. Med. J.*, **218**, 474

Golding, A. M. B. and Tosey, D. (1980). The cost of high technology medicine. *Lancet*, **2**, 195

4

Chronic renal failure in the United Kingdom: referral, funding and staffing
Roger Gabriel

In many parts of the country facilities for dialysis are inadequate (Editorial, 1981a). They are lamentably poor for patients with renal failure over the age of 60 years and for diabetics in renal failure.

4.1 SOURCES OF PATIENTS FOR DIALYSIS OR TRANSPLANTATION

The majority of renal physicians work as tertiary physicians, their patients being referred to them by consultant colleagues. A minority of patients are referred by general practitioners for assessment and treatment. About half the people aged up to 50 years receive treatment for terminal renal failure. Those who die without dialysis have either been referred for a renal opinion and considered unsuitable or have never been referred or referred too late. In addition some patients may present to a general medical firm in terminal decompensated renal failure and die before expert aid can be summoned.

The Medical Services Study Group of the Royal College of Physicians (1981) presented brief details of 53 out of 122 patients all under the age of 50 years with terminal renal failure who were considered unsuitable for dialysis. The validity and relevance of the analysis was questioned (Editorial, 1981b; Cameron *et al.*, 1981; Large and Ahmad, 1981; Michael and Adu, 1981; Parsons and Lock, 1981; Verwilghen, 1981). Nevertheless the 53 untreated people did have the advantage of a specialist opinion. What is not known with any precision is the number of patients who might prove suitable for dialysis but never have the benefit of a renal consultation. I estimate that about 25–30 patients per million of population per annum fall into this category. About 40 new cases of chronic renal failure occur per million of population per annum up to the age of 50 years. If older age groups are included, the incidence of chronic renal failure increases to perhaps more than 60 new patients per million per annum. Since only 24 patients per million of population per annum currently receive treatment (Jacobs *et al.*, 1981) the estimate of 25–30 untreated patients per annum per million of population is probably conservative. The population of Great Britain is approximately 56 million and hence the annual number of untreated patients is of the order of 1400 to 1700. This estimate includes potential patients up to the age of 70 years.

Until it is recognized that treatment may be available for at least a proportion of these patients, they will not be referred for possible treatment. In some medical circles the elderly (people over the age of 65 or 70 years) are not considered for active treatment (other than drug therapy) of a chronic disease. Thus the thought of referral does not arise. In any general medical clinic the number of patients possibly requiring dialysis is small, and therefore a consultant in general medicine can only have limited experience in renal medicine and may not have established channels of referral to a renal unit. Conversely, renal physicians may have been dilatory in offering their services to colleagues in their Region: medicine is a conservative profession.

4.2 MONEY NECESSARY TO EXPAND DIALYSIS IN THE UNITED KINGDOM

It is probable that the deficiency in patient referral will be resolved. The number of dialysis patients in this country is slowly increasing and the rate of increase will accelerate as continuous ambulatory peritoneal dialysis (CAPD) becomes more widely applied. However, the probability of extra DHSS funds being made available to pay for the envisaged expansion is not great. The cost of the fabric and equipment of a new 10-station Regional hospital haemodialysis unit was estimated at £350000 (1979 prices) (*Hansard*, 1981). Not only will current renal units have to deal with an expanding number of patients but, until a fool-proof method is devised for connecting CAPD dialysis fluid to the patient line, an increasing proportion of renal in-patient beds will be occupied by patients receiving treatment for bacterial peritonitis.

The difficulties associated with treating more patients without any increase in the number of available beds will increase in the next few years. Described below are five possible ways whereby the expected enlarged population of dialysis patients may be managed without major additional expense.

4.2.1 Minimal care units for haemodialysis

Not many such units exist in Britain but they are economical to run and save the patients' time and travelling costs. There seems no obvious reason why minimal care units could not be shared by patients originating from different Regional units.

4.2.2 District General Hospital CAPD units

Some District General Hospitals remote from Regional units could be equipped to treat their own (and neighbouring) patients with terminal renal failure. Regional renal units could train staff from the District General Hospital who would then return and treat their own patients. Regular liaison with the Regional unit would be needed. Given goodwill and enthusiasm such schemes would be feasible and for many patients, particularly the older ones, travelling would be reduced and they could perhaps, benefit from the sense of community which exists in many District General Hospitals. The topic has been discussed more fully elsewhere (Gabriel, 1982). CAPD dialysis fluid costs about £5000 per annum (1982 prices) per patient. The total cost for one person over a 12 month period would perhaps be £6500 – the extra £1500 covering the cost of admissions, the catheters, antibiotics and cleansing solutions. If this money were available from District General Hospital funds it might permit the expansion of national regional facilities without apparently affecting the total renal bill. Currently Regional renal units are financed directly by money via Region from the DHSS, so that the expenses of renal units are paid independently of the general hospital in which they are situated.

4.2.3 Transplant coordinators

More need to be appointed. One important function of such people would be to impress on hospital staff who send patients for dialysis that the hospital medical staff have a responsibility to obtain cadaver kidneys.

4.2.4 Live donors

Intensive efforts should be made to seek live donors among the close relatives of patients in renal failure.

4.2.5 Private sector finance

There are only three private dialysis units in Britain; all are in London and presumably cater for a transient international population of patients. While the present government indicated that it would like 25% of medical and surgical conditions to be dealt with in the private sector it does not appear likely that chronic dialysis could easily be set into that financial context. Medical insurance cover for chronic renal failure could be established but small numbers of patients who are scattered across the country make the siting of private dialysis units very difficult to plan.

The above suggestions, probably with the exception of the expansion of the private sector, could allow greater numbers of patients with terminal renal failure to obtain treatment. In essence the individual patient should spend less time in the Regional unit be he transferred to home dialysis, transplanted or managed on CAPD from a District General Hospital.

4.3 STAFFING OF RENAL UNITS

Dialysis is almost exclusively a nursing procedure. Medical staff play a minor role in the management of chronic dialysis patients. Unfortunately, there is a continuous lack of nurses in the majority of British hospital wards. If the expected increase in numbers of patients for renal replacement therapy occurs then the majority of these patients (who will be amongst the older age groups) will need to be taught to dialyse themselves. Technical and practical advice and psychological support would be available from a telephone call to the supervising unit.

It is debatable whether renal unit nurses are in shorter supply than are nurses for other specialized areas. It may be that because only a minority of British hospitals have renal units staff nurses do not develop the idea of specializing in renal nursing. Student and pupil nurses in those hospitals with renal units only gain a very superficial idea of renal work and may therefore never think of working within this discipline. Perhaps fears of hepatitis B still have a detrimental effect upon recruitment. For some, the psychological demands of longterm care of renal patients is daunting compared with the smaller degree and shorter duration of involvement with patients in general wards.

In the last decade, there has been an expansion of specialized units and any nurse wishing to gain experience in a special unit has a number from which to choose.

It is clearly improbable that many more nurses will be available to staff renal units in Britain in the future. Perhaps there is hope that satellite or minimal care units, which by definition require smaller numbers of less highly trained nursing staff, will be able to carry some of the load currently undertaken by Regional units. If District General Hospital CAPD units do develop, then demands upon Regional units should stabilize if not actually fall.

4.4 CONCLUSIONS

In Britain less than half the possible population of dialysis patients are at present receiving treatment. This poor record should improve as it is realized that facilities for older patients are available. An increase in patients will require more money to buy materials. If the CAPD population were primarily increased the additional cost in 1982 per patient per annum would be about £6500. If a number of District General Hospitals undertook CAPD the extra expense might be carried from non-renal funds. It is improbable that the numbers of renal nurses will increase. Therefore it is necessary that as far as possible every patient pass through his renal unit as quickly as possible. To offer treatment to more patients with terminal renal failure, home haemodialysis, CAPD and grafting will need to be more efficiently supplied than at present so as to use the relatively fixed resources of the NHS to the best possible advantage.

References

Cameron, S., Chantler, C., Haycock, G., Ogg, C. S., Williams, D. G., Jones, N., Hilton, P. J. and Wing, A. J. (1981). Audit in renal failure. *Br. Med. J.*, **283**, 555

Editorial (1981a). Ethics and the nephrologist. *Lancet,* **1**, 594

Editorial (1981b). Audit in renal failure: the wrong target? *Br. Med. J.*, **283**, 261

Gabriel, R. (1982). Renal failure - dilemma and developments. *Br. Med. J.*, **284**, 1406

Hansard (1981). **Col. 1350,** 30th April

Jacobs, C., Broyer, M., Brunner, F.P., Brynger, H., Donckerwolcke, R.S., Kramer, P., Selwood, N.H., Wing, A.J. and Blake, P.H. (1981). Combined report on regular dialysis and transplantation in Europe, XI, 1980. *Proc. Eur. Dial. Transplant Assoc.*, **18,** 2

Large, B and Ahmad, R. (1981). Audit in renal failure. *Br. Med. J.,* **283,** 556

Medical Services Study Group of the Royal College of Physicians. (1981). Deaths from chronic renal failure under the age of 50. *Br. Med. J.,* **283,** 283

Michael, J. and Adu, D. (1981). Audit in renal failure. *Br. Med. J.,* **283,** 556

Parsons, V. and Lock, P.M. (1981). Audit and renal failure. *Br. Med. J.,* **283,** 556

Verwilghen, R.L. (1981). Audit in renal failure. *Br. Med. J.,* **283,** 556

5

The selection and de-selection of patients for dialysis and transplantation
V. Parsons and P. M. Lock

5.1 INTRODUCTION

Any modern society should be judged among other aspects, by the way in which its sick and handicapped are cared for and assisted. That is an issue of public policy that no-one can ultimately escape (Maxwell, 1981). However, no country irrespective of its wealth can supply its population with all the types of treatment that medical science has the potential to offer. It has been a matter for central and local policy in the UK that the treatment of renal failure should expand slowly as far as hospital-based renal units and dialysis facilities are concerned (Renal Association,1976), in the hope that transplantation, a cheaper form of treatment, would in time care increasingly for those who need renal replacement therapy (Pincherle, 1977) thereby avoiding the massive increase in dialysis facilities which has occurred in the majority of European countries.

The acceptance of this slow, often pragmatic, expansion by the medical profession and national and regional planners indicates how decisions of who to treat rest on economic availability rather than on clinical issues (*Lancet* Leader, 1981). Two independent pieces of data have highlighted the problems of non-treatment that physicians and nephrologists have been facing. The first is the striking increase in the number of patients placed on continuous ambulatory peritoneal dialysis (CAPD), reflecting a hitherto untapped pool of untreated patients (Jacobs *et al.*, 1981). The second was a review of patients under 50 dying with end-stage renal failure in a population of over six million, who were untreated despite the fact that the nephrologists concerned denied any shortage of facilities (Medical Services Study Group, 1981). These data provoked criticism of the selection procedures which were obviously, in the first example, denying treatment to patients now on CAPD and in the second example denying consideration of some patients for any form of treatment (*British Medical Journal* Leader, 1981; Cameron *et al.*, 1981; *Times* Leader, 1981).

5.2 SOME ISSUES IN SELECTION

With the advent of longterm dialysis, various criteria for selection have been used (Fox, 1981). Initially, the young uncomplicated patient with a good record of stable relationships and possibly a home to dialyse in, was selected in preference to the older patient with complicated disease, who had no regular employment and lived on his own in a property unsuitable for dialysis. This enabled a high patient survival rate to be achieved, and, for the treatment, be it dialysis or transplantation, to be seen as relatively successful; even more so in fact than the treatment for the commonest

Table 5.1   Reasons given for rejection

Taylor *et al.*, 1975	Parsons and Lock, 1980
Age	Age
Heart disease	Psychiatric illness
Psychiatric illness	Hepatitis
Blindness	Social situation
Type of renal disease	Blindness in a diabetic
Other complicating disease	
Annual income	
Sex	

cancers where there has never been any comment on the selection of patients for therapy (Knapp, 1982).

As selection criteria expanded, various clinicians reported (or more often didn't report) patients whom they felt unable to help medically, on grounds other than the general criterion of excluding those over 60 years of age (Table 5.1).

Two studies have reported the variety of response and lack of conformity among nephrologists, the first (Taylor *et al.*, 1975) used 100 real and simulated cases, reviewed by eight clinicians, and the second (Parsons and Lock, 1980) 40 simulated patients reviewed by 25 physicians; the differences and similarities between these are shown in Table 5.2.

Table 5.2   Unsuitable patients

	1969–72 London N.E.	1968–70 N. Ireland	1970–79 London K.C.H.	1978–79 Tri-Region
Patients	1260	222	458	676
Unsuitable	288 (23%)	46 (21%)	22 (5%)	53 (8%)
Psychosocial	67	17	4	13
Medical complications	123	15	8	15
Diabetes	20	14	6	17
Australia antigen + ve	4	0	2	0
Died waiting	74	–	2	8

Both real and simulated situations reveal a variety of priorities which come into play, not only for the individual patient presenting at a time of restricted facilities, but which exist independently of economic limitations and reflect physicians' attitudes to the patients they would wish to choose for treatment.

5.2.1   Age

One of the highest discriminating factors is age, which carries within it an increasing number of complicating medical conditions and a decreasing possibility of potential benefit. Age counted in years is not a valid measurement alone, and the flat refusal to treat patients over a certain chronological age denies a quite reasonable existence to a proportion of patients, and, more fundamentally, denies human rights which are not age-dependent (Leenan, 1979).

Various surveys have been carried out in patients aged 50–80 and in some centres a quarter of the patients now accepted are over the age of 65. Haemodialysis extended life in the majority for nearly 2 years which can be expressed as an increase of 16% in their life span. Neither age itself nor the number of years beyond 70 can be a predictor of survival, although the presence of hypertension and gastrointestinal haemorrhage carry a worse prognosis (Chester *et al.*, 1979).

5.2.2 Psychiatric illness

All series of actual and simulated patients contain a proportion rejected on psychiatric grounds. In our simulated series three patients had difficulty being accepted with diagnoses of schizophrenia, drug addiction and a long history of mental illness. In the report of the Medical Services Study Group (1981), 11 patients out of a total of 122 dying of renal failure, with and without treatment, were said to have mental subnormality, psychosis, suicide or chronic depression. In the Glasgow study (Taylor *et al.*, 1975) seven of the eight allocating physicians put psychiatric causes in the list of significant predictors of rejection, though one did not. The problem lies in determining at the time of referral whether the mental illness has any metabolic basis which would be reversed with treatment. If the mental illness and disability predates any signs of renal failure, then the chances are that it will influence the prognosis of the patient on dialysis or following transplantation (Farmer *et al.*, 1979).

Our own attitude is to give patients a trial of therapy to see how they are affected, and whether they manage to adapt once the metabolic abnormality is removed. Clearly, the withdrawal of therapy if their mental condition deteriorates, as it does occasionally to the stage of dementia, is difficult. Our own psychiatrists have resisted pressures to detain and treat such patients against their will if they refuse to co-operate once treatment has been started, even if they are suffering from severe depression or frank psychotic illness. A second problem is highlighted by the two patients considered by Fox (1981); their mental condition was irreversible as the result of progressive organic cerebral damage secondary to either metabolic or vascular disease. Under these circumstances further therapy only compounds their suffering and can legally be withdrawn.

5.2.3 Social considerations

With a shortage of dialysis places in hospital and an insufficient supply of kidneys for transplantation, the solitary, homeless, untransplantable patient is made permanently dependent on hospital facilities, and hence at a disadvantage when these are limited and confined to those who can be trained for self treatment which releases facilities for newcomers. With an expansion of CAPD and satellite self-care dialysis facilities, the objection to this type of patient should be overcome. Similarly, non-English speaking patients cannot justifiably be denied treatment on this basis alone; they are difficult but certainly not impossible to train, as many large city units have shown. These and other social considerations based on issues of sex, intelligence and moral values may present special difficulties, but cannot be legitimate grounds for exclusion and it is to be hoped that such criteria will disappear.

5.2.4 Medical exclusions

One of the problems facing modern medicine is the decision to cease treatment, or not to correct abnormalities complicating diseases with a poor prognosis. This applies to renal failure complicating terminal illnesses such as carcinoma, irreversible liver failure and advanced cerebro- and cardiovascular disease. The very use of life-preserving measures prolongs suffering and does not allow the patient to die with dignity or choice. Where such decisions have been tested in the courts, as in the case where the patient was a ward of the state and incompetent to express his own wishes, the non-use of distressing and hazardous treatment was legally upheld in two courts (McIntyre, 1981).

Any policy that does not involve rejection on medical grounds inevitably leads to the acceptance of patients with complicating diseases which lead to more difficulties and disabilities than can be treated by dialysis or transplantation; thus the patient with advanced malignant disease can be rescued from ·uraemia only to suffer the sequelae of metastatic disease. The same applies to the patient with advanced vascular disease as typified by the diabetic with vascular complications requiring sequential amputations until vascular access via the limbs has become impossible. There seems to be little disagreement about such situations as, despite dialysis and transplantation, sepsis and anorexia take their toll.

A particularly worrying complication is that of hepatitis, due, in a majority of patients, to Australia antigen associated infections. These patients are often excluded from the normal dialysis facilities in renal units, and, if they present with hepatitis rather than contract it during treatment, this will act as a strong discriminant against their selection. However, hepatitis is mysteriously absent as a cause for rejection in some large series, and it must be recognized as influencing patient referral, since these patients are often listed as died waiting for the elective treatment of transplantation. Comments made at a symposium five years ago, stating that such patients have a slim chance of acceptance in the majority of units (Robinson, 1978), still apply. Their management carries risks to the staff, and, if segregation is not possible, to other patients as well, something which the majority of staff still see as unacceptable. The answer lies in the provision of segregated accommodation and separate staff who are willing to take the extra care and precautions which will enable these patients to be dialysed and, ideally, quickly transplanted. Only a minority of these patients progress to liver damage and to deny treatment to the majority is a serious indictment of our facilities.

5.3   WHO SHOULD TAKE PART IN THE DECISION-MAKING PROCESS?

One of the concerns that the recent Reith Lectures highlighted was the way doctors as a profession kept the decision-making process to themselves, and acted as judge and jury, denying patients the right to know the issues involved (Kennedy, 1981). Where the decisions are based solely on medical criteria, then more than one or two physicians or surgeons should be involved to ensure that decisions are made with a full discussion of the present state of the art. Where decisions are made on other than medical criteria, then they should involve those qualified to express an opinion and the patient and his family so that they may act on the informed views of experts, challenge decisions and, if necessary, seek alternative opinions (Leenan, 1982). In our hospital group, working in a bankrupt position, decisions were taken by the administration, who wanted these to be conveyed by physicians, arguing that the profession is used to delivering bad prognoses and could best soften and disguise rejections based on economics, avoiding undue upset to the patient. Such methods are both a betrayal of trust and a misuse of the physician's role, and should, as de Wardener (1980) has stated, be forced back to the administration. If facilities are temporarily full or exhausted patients must be told to seek help in another dialysis area that has spare capacity, as obtains in other disciplines of medicine.

To obviate late referral which may force a hurried choice of treatment, more physicians with an interest in renal medicine are needed in general hospitals, a point stressed by Knapp (1982). It is harder to reject a patient whom one has cared for over a long period, planned a fistula, followed through the progression of his disease, and with whom one has discussed future provision in the relative calm of the consulting room. Here personal interest is matched by personal responsibility and facilities can be anticipated and planned for. While administrative authorities fail to acknowledge that the 40 patients per million of population who present with renal failure each year need to be matched, in a pool of 400 patients per million, who are actually on treatment, with the 10 per million who leave this pool each year, provision of care for those with renal failure will remain inadequate.

On the professional side must come an increasing willingness to think of organ donation and to make the process more accurate and less worrying for the relatives. The majority of the profession are in favour of transplantation and yet the proportion of kidneys retrieved out of those available is still too small to meet the increasing waiting list. The advent of transplant co-ordinators and a possible change in the law are ways forward (Calne, 1982).

References

Calne, R. Y. (1982). Whatever happened to charity? *Br. Med. J.*, **284**, 998

Cameron, S. C., Chantler, C., Haycock, G., Ogg, C. S., Williams, D. G., Jones, N., Hilton, P. J. and Wing, A. J. (1981). Audit in renal failure. *Br. Med. J.*, **283**, 555

Chester, A. C., Rakowski, T. A. and Argy, W. P. (1979). Haemodialysis in the eighth and ninth decades of life. *Arch. Intern. Med.*, **139**, 1001

Farmer, C. J., Bewick, M., Parsons, V. and Snowden, S. A. (1979). Survival on home haemodialysis: its relationship with physical symptomatology, psycho-social background and psychiatric morbidity. *Psychol. Med.*, **9**, 515

Fox, R. C. (1981). Exclusion for dialysis. A sociologic and legal perspective. *Kidney Int.*, **19**, 139

Jacobs, C., Broyer, M., Brunner, F.P., Brynger, H., Donckerwolcke, R. A., Kramer, P., Selwood, N. H., Wing, A. J. and Blake, B. H. (1981). Combined report on regular dialysis and transplantation in Europe, XI, 1980 *Proc. Eur. Dial. Transplant Assoc.*, **18**, 38

Kennedy, I. (1981). *The Last Taboo in the Unmasking of Medicine,* Chapter 7. (London: Allen & Unwin)

Knapp, M. S. (1982). Renal failure: dilemmas and developments. *Br. Med. J.*, **284**, 847

Leader (1981). Audit in renal failure: the wrong target. *Br. Med. J.*, **283**, 261

Leader (1981). Ethics and the nephrologist. *Lancet*, **1**, 594

Leader (1981). The statistics of life and hope. *Times*, **July 24**, 15

Leenan, H. J. J. (1979). The selection of patients in the event of a scarcity of medical facilities. *Int. J. Med. Law.*, **2**, 161

Leenan, H. J. J. (1982). Selection of patients. *J. Med. Ethics*, **8**, 33

Maxwell, R. J. (1981). *Health and Wealth: An International Study of Health Care Spending* (Aldershot: Lexington Books)

Medical Services Study Group of the Royal College of Physicians, (1981). Deaths from chronic renal failure under the age of 50. *Br. Med. J.*, **283**, 283

McIntyre, K. M. (1981). Recent case law and medical life and death decision making. *Ala. J. Med. Sci.*, **18**, 381

Parsons, V. and Lock, P. M. (1980). Triage and the patient with renal failure. *J. Med. Ethics*, **6**, 173

Pincherle, G. (1977). Services for patients with chronic renal failure in England and Wales. *Health Trends*, **9**, 41

Renal Association Executive (1976). Distributions of nephrological services for adults in Great Britain. *Br. Med. J.*, **2**, 903

Robinson, B. H. B. (1978). Selection of patients for dialysis and transplantation. In Anderson, J. L., Parsons F. M. and Jones, D. E. (eds.). *Living with Renal Failure*. pp. 9–18. (Lancaster: MTP Press)

Taylor, T. R., Aitchison, J., Parker, L. S. and Moore, M. R. (1975). Individual differences in selecting patients for regular haemodialysis. *Br. Med. J.*, **2**, 380

de Wardener, H. E. (1980). Psychological and socio-economic aspects of dialysis and transplantation. *Proc. Eur. Dial. Transplant Assoc.*, **17**, 519

Discussion

R. Gabriel (St Mary's Hospital, London): Why has the Department of Health been so dilatory in producing the very thinnest analysis of what has been labelled as expensive treatment? I am impressed by the paucity of Dr Pincherle's data.

Pincherle: These are only preliminary results.

Gabriel: Dialysis has been available for 15–20 years!

Cattell: The point is well taken. We are all aware that we have been asking for some years about the costs of this treatment. There has been a great requirement to find out just what it is costing us.

Pincherle: That is very true. On the other hand, hernias have been treated for some two hundred years and no one can give me the cost of treating a hernia.

T. D. Clarke (Yorkshire Regional Health Authority): I was somewhat intrigued by Dr Gabriel's suggestion that CAPD patients should somehow be lost in District General Hospitals. There are a great many heavy burdens, new burdens, on the drug bill – I speak as a pharmacist – such as total parenteral nutrition and the ever-increasing use of cytotoxic agents. Dr Gabriel's suggestion would to some extent be counter-productive, because when the moneys are worked out and when our bright new teams come into being and start to examine every halfpenny, they will only allow a very small quantity of money for the patients on CAPD and we may not get as much as we would like.

Gabriel: I did not expand the concept of introducing CAPD into District General Hospitals because of time. I do not suggest that such people are abandoned in District General Hospitals. I would suggest that a free and regular interchange of people between the Regional renal unit and the District General Hospital concerned be set up so that staff working in both units would get to know each other, the Regional unit could train the local people and the Regional unit would be available for telephonic advice. Perhaps the Regional unit's renal physician should do monthly clinics or something like that. Cytotoxics and total parenteral nutrition are expensive, *but*, because the sums of money for renal units come direct from Region, it

49

may be that the money that goes to District General Hospitals comes from a different pocket. If a physician or surgeon in a District General Hospital picks up a syringe full of some expensive drug which, in his clinical opinion is appropriate for the patient, he may use it. Presumably, therefore if a physician picks up litres and litres of peritoneal dialysis fluid in the District General Hospital, he may use it also.

We should not be too obsessed with money. It is only NHS money! It is not proper money. Real money is the stuff in our hip pockets.

R. Gokal (Manchester Royal Infirmary): I would like to take up the point about the use of CAPD in District General Hospitals. The idea is certainly appealing. In Manchester we are looking into this and already beginning to evolve a liaison with District General Hospitals to try to spread the workload. That has to be the aim, rather than to deploy CAPD or renal replacement therapy entirely at the District level. Currently CAPD has a high complication rate and those of us who feel we know about CAPD still record disastrous results. If we are to try and deploy this treatment entirely at District General Hospital level it will bounce back at us even more seriously.

There is a place for co-ordinated action. We are looking into this seriously and will be starting to implement it. Staffing must be co-ordinated. No one can run a unit without adequate staffing. If there is to be Regional involvement at the District General Hospital level then there has to be a complete range of staff and expertise available at the District General Hospital. This will mean the appointment of a physician with an interest in renal disease to produce a renal base which can co-ordinate with the super-specialized unit. If that sort of set up can be made available we shall run a successful service.

That, of course, comes back to the fact that we just do not have enough renal units. In the North-West Region there are three renal units serving a population of 5 000 000 all grouped in Manchester. We have patients spending their entire day to-ing and fro-ing hundreds of miles between home and renal unit to see us for 10 or 15 minutes. It is to minimize this, to make life more tolerable for the patient, that we need to expand, but the expansion will need to come by deployment of extra units and extra facilities in the District General Hospitals.

Cattell: What is being suggested is 'satellite' dialysis with District General Hospitals practising CAPD. Is there anyone present who has such experience within the United Kingdom?

H. Lupton (East Birmingham Hospital): At Hereford, Dr Ross looks after a considerable number of our patients who live in his area. It is a long way to our hospital for outpatient visits and he does the major part of the outpatient care. If the patients develop complications such as peritonitis, he can treat them in his own hospital.

He has no formal renal unit but we do have good telephone connections.

A. I. Murphy (Southend and District Association for Kidney Care): We are actually doing what is being discussed now. We have persuaded, pressured and collected money to set up CAPD treatment in our local general hospital, and we have persuaded other people to give us money to set up a minimal care satellite dialysis unit. So, based on Southend General Hospital we have a renal unit in the community and it is working.

But, more importantly, we are coming to a watershed because we can only raise enough money yearly to treat four or five patients; all are in the 60-plus age group. They have been turned down by everybody else but we still think they are worth saving. So what do we do know? I have started negotiations for joint funding and I have already got a 'no, no' response. Our new District Health Authority has said that financial cuts are in progress and I think we could be one of the services that may be cut. It is all very well to say that the District General Hospital will give us money; they would not even give us the money to start. They told us to go away, we were wasting our time. But we do not think we are. How do we go about it from now on?

Cattell: What Mrs Murphy is saying is that Southend General Hospital is deselecting for them!

V. Parsons: I think her unit is in grave difficulties. But we believe that we have both freedom of speech and freedom of access. If patients who are already on dialysis are likely to be turned down, this is a very very sad issue and one that should be taken straight to the ombudsman. There is no argument about that.

If there are patients who as yet are not on treatment but who might need treatment, then it would be worth writing to the nearby renal units. There is a splendid unit at Cambridge and there is a unit in Brighton that has never turned down a patient of ours from London. I know that it is hard for patients to travel, and to have to tell someone that in order to stay alive he/she may have to move home and house. That may be so. But I do ask those who have patients in need to write round to as many renal units as they can. In our experience there is usually someone somewhere who will say yes, but it may not be in the local area. This is the problem of very strict budgets and it is really a national problem.

Pryor: I can assure Mrs Murphy that if her association contacts us in Norwich we shall be very helpful. We are in the process of trying to set up satellite units ourselves, using a computerized system. If Southend approaches us I am sure we shall be able to help.

G. T. Taylor (Norfolk and Norwich Hospital): Dr Bone, from Liverpool, at the Stirling meeting (Bone, 1978), outlined the way in which satellite units could be set up, and since that meeting Merseyside has established four functioning satellite units. Three of them are on an inner ring with minimal staff and support the patients on three days of the week in two sessions. More recently an outer ring of satellite units has started to evolve with even less staff, or perhaps no staff at all, except for some who commute from the main unit. Patients in the outer ring are assisted by either a partner or a dialysis friend.

The fourth unit which is situated in the outer ring, and which may already have opened, is some 50 or 60 miles from the central unit and will rely heavily on the support of local physicians, although they will obviously refer some things to the central unit.

Cattell: We are talking about satellite units and minimal care units, and also about the use of District General Hospitals for CAPD. Are those rings of units within hospital precincts? Are they staffed by the parent renal unit? Who funds them?

Taylor: It was found convenient to negotiate through the Area Health Authority and to use property that was owned by the Health Authority. The first unit is situated in a psycho-geriatric hospital. The second unit is in a cottage hospital, previously used by surgeons but now used solely by general practitioners; the operating theatre was converted into a dialysis unit. The third unit was sited in a hospital which had virtually closed and would probably have been condemned had it not been put to dialysis use. The fourth unit is within the grounds of a hospital using a portacabin that has been specially installed for dialysis use.

A fifth unit is also within an existing hospital, using a converted ward for dialysis.

Cattell: Who staffs and funds them?

Taylor: Mostly through the Health Authorities. One of them has been funded via a donation from industry for a number of years, and the cost is due to be taken over by the Region.

F. M. Parsons: Our friends from London are talking utter rubbish. Let me refer back to the Figure [Figure 4, Chapter 1] on the productivity of continental units. We are talking here in the UK of one dialysis centre per million of population, each looking after approximately 61 patients. France is providing 3.5 centres per million of population or therabouts. These are proper units not satellites.

Let us appreciate that we must achieve an intake of 40 new patients or therabouts per million of population per year. Satellite units and part-time physicians cannot cope with this work. What we have got to do is to persuade the Department of Health that we must double the number of dialysis centres. This applies not just to haemodialysis but CAPD as well.

In travelling up and down the country I have seen units setting up CAPD on shoestrings. I was in one that was using a general medical ward. The untrained junior nursing staff were administering CAPD. This is what I was getting at in Chapter 1. I want an answer out of the Department of Health within a month.

According to my estimates, for every 12 patients on CAPD an additional senior member of the nursing staff is required. She is the home administrator, she is the social worker and she is the person who has to care for that patient. If we are having a fantastic drop-out on CAPD, this is because we as renal physicians are working on a shoestring. We are not training our patients properly, which means we are not looking after our patients properly. We should no be talking about satellite units until we have doubled our dialysis units.

Gabriel: In *Hansard* in 1980 the cost of the fabric and equipment of a 10-bedded Regional dialysis unit was stated to be £350 000. That was to set it up which is relatively cheap. But it takes nurses to run the unit. Medical staff are cheap and that is easy, but nurses are more difficult to recruit. I apologise to my friends from north of London but I am not totally in agreement with their views. It is for this sort of reason that my thoughts some months ago went towards District General Hospitals. I know they are busy but CAPD could be slotted into their duties. I do not think it realistic to go to the Department and ask for additional renal units, either for the capital cost, or, if we could recruit them, for the salaries of nursing staff.

Cattell: Let me take this up in context of the relationship between the number of patients being treated in a particular country and the Gross National Product of that country [see Chapter 2, Figure 1]. Let us not argue about how to calculate the Gross National Product, but there we are, bang on the line. There are other countries above us and some below us. The interpretation by the EDTA leaves a great deal to be desired. I could suggest that the first answer to our problem is to persuade our colleagues to make more money for the country. Perhaps we should address ourselves to the Confederation of British Industries and the Trades Union Conference in that every time there is a strike another guy loses dialysis because we as a nation are not making enough money. Perhaps we are getting the service that is appropriate to a poor country. Of course that graph says nothing about how efficiently the money is used. Unlike Frank Parsons I think it is quite unrealistic to believe that there will suddenly be a vast increase in the amount of money available for health care, out of which the money for dialysis must come.

I also disagree with Vic Parsons in that I do not think we can shrug it off and tell the Department that they must redistribute the money for health care. We as clinicians have got a lot to do with this. We need to examine the use of money – are we effective?

If I wish to be really provocative, which I do, I would suggest that we take a look at various other sectors of health care. If we had a dictate from the

Department of Health tomorrow which said that all cases of abdominal cancer beyond a certain degree would not be operated on we would generate a vast amount of money for our hospitals. If we went round our hospitals and examined why patients were in hospital as opposed to being at home with their families, we could, I suspect, throw out some 60% of the patients in acute stay hospitals.

I agree that there is a desperate need for more money for this immensely successful form of treatment. I do not believe for half a second that a vast amount of money will suddenly be thrown at us. We, the profession, have got to examine how we can generate that money from within ourselves. My interest in pursuing the question of satellite units is that around the environs of Westminster this is called the art of the possible. One starts off with a little thin wedge and drives it bigger, and bigger, and bigger, and bigger until all these extra units are functional. We do not believe that suddenly anyone will give us anything for anything. When dialysis started in Britain it took months and months and months of hammering away, using, for example, the media and demonstrating to society that to refuse to accept renal replacement was wholly irresponsible.

P. Mancini (DHSS): This is not a question but a clarification. I have been hearing mumblings about our costings and the fact that those for CAPD seem to be based on three patients only. In fact that is not correct. The complications data relate only to three patients in the sample. The basic costing information relates to about 20 CAPD patients in the unit chosen. That is a bit harder.

Gabriel: It is still very very thin.

Mancini: It is thin, but it was a random sample taken under very severe time constraints; three hospitals in six months. If we can get more economists we can do more work.

B. M. Reed (Dulwich Hospital): Unit directors are the first to point out that units are understaffed and yet all directors adopt a policy of re-using disposable dialysers. This is time-consuming for all the staff. Nurses and technicians become very despondent because of the time they must spend on re-using, teaching patients to re-use and talking to patients about why they should re-use a disposable dialyser. No patient comes to the unit director or to the consultants to ask these questions. It is the technicians and the nursing staff who must spend their time answering them. Directors of units should try to adopt a policy of disposing of disposables and then unit staff will be able to do a lot more of the work that they should be doing.

Cattell: I am told by Prof. Pryor that he does not re-use. We certainly do, and it is time-consuming and so on. The workload can be reduced by automating it. There is no reason for manual re-use. There is equipment available; one plugs in and it is done automatically.

Reed: But the nurses, the technicians and the staff have to go and plug in the machine and they have to return when the machine is finished. It is still time-consuming – more so than some realize. Dr Cattell is suggesting that it takes no time but this is not so. In most of the units that I have been to I have seen staff discussing disposable dialysers, working on the new units, repairing them, talking to home patients about it. These things tend not to be taken into account.

Cattell: I entirely take the point. It is time-consuming. Our reason for re-using is absolutely straightforward. We have a fixed budget allocated to us each year to sustain our global programme. At the moment we are moving to using disposable equipment but there is absolutely no way that we could fund out of our budget the single use of disposable items. We re-use both dialysers and lines. If we were to go over to single use we would have to cut the number of patients on regular dialysis treatment by 25%.

Gabriel: Would it be feasible to pull the wool over the eyes of those who control the money so that if dialysis fluid for CAPD were bought in District General Hospitals it would come from a different budget? Is that a feasible ploy?

Pincherle: It all depends on how the region does its budgeting, and this varies from Region to Region. Some renal units have their own budget which is allocated to them. In other instances that is not the case. What is true is that there is a fixed amount of money for the Region and it is up to the region to decide how it is allocated. If a District General Hospital were to introduce a significant amount of CAPD from a fixed budget then, for that District, something else would have to go, and that is something that has to be decided by the District.

Whilst we are on the question of CAPD and District General Hospitals, I should like to emphasize the importance of ensuring that the staff who look after this are fully trained. There have been cases where hospitals have started CAPD with incompletely trained staff. This brings the whole service into disrepute and is to be deplored.

Gabriel: I agree entirely.

Cattell: I think I can answer Dr Gabriel's question from bitter experience. Yes, you can get away with it. You can get away with concealing your CAPD requirements, your fluid and so forth, within the general compost of a District General Hospital's activity for a limited period of time. Then suddenly the pharmacist will turn round and ask why the hospital is buying so much dialysing fluid – and then the cat will be out of the bag. And they get very tense about it.

D. G. Oreopoulos (University of Toronto): Are the reasons for the rejection of patients cited by Vic Parsons a cover-up of a conscious or subconscious conviction of those who refuse so that society can spend the money more profitably on a larger number of healthy older or younger patients?

V. Parsons: Yes, I think that is so in one sense, and I am analysing my own feelings. We looked at what other nephrologists said. Some said that this was a very difficult and painful exercise and they were very distressed by it. They obviously had the feeling that if they had to choose between a young person and an older person they would choose the younger person. That is one fact.

Secondly, there is still, in British nephrology, a hard core of nephrologists who trained before dialysis existed. We do know that over the years they have advised the DHSS because they are very senior people. There has been a feeling among them that dialysis is not what nephrologists should be doing. In other words, it is a job for 'plumbers'. This feeling carries over.

Prof Oreopoulos has picked on it here, rather sadly. There are still physicians of some seniority, nephrologists perhaps of some seniority too, who feel that the vast expenditure on dialysis is not matched by an equal expenditure on research into renal disease, hypertension, or whatever.

Recently Parliament was told that just under £1 million a year is spent on research into renal diseases in the UK. That compares very poorly with what is spent in Canada and the US. There is a lobby that says it should be cured rather than treated. That comes through in the discussion about age. If the patient is already sadly ill there is no sense in prolonging that suffering! The British pragmatic approach, the more patients the more sweat and the more agony, is to be compared with the US where the more patients treated the bigger the income for the unit. If we could have £5000 for every patient treated per year the figures in this country would soon rise, because it could mean more staff, more social workers, more CAPD. When that happens these reasons should change. I hope so.

M. Boulton-Jones (Glasgow Royal Infirmary): I moved from London to Glasgow just after a survey was taken and I would agree that the gentlemen in London have it easy compared to our problems in Glasgow. The lists of reasons for rejecting patients express the places available. Nevertheless, it is incumbent on us all to put on political pressure to increase the number of facilities. The number of units should be doubled and they should be started in areas of scarcity.

However, we have to make the best of our own facilities. The advent of CAPD enabled us to take on more patients. It was very interesting that at that point, when we were taking on every patient who was referred, it was still only about 25 per million per year. The refusal rate was not at nephrologist level but because the referring units and hospitals had all learnt their behaviour from the days of scarcity. We had to write round all the units in the West of Scotland and we have now raised the intake rate to roughly 30 per million per year. But there are many blocks to be unplugged.

Pryor: We find the same figures in Norwich. A lot of people are either trying to be kind to us by not exposing us to these difficult decisions, or they themselves are not fully aware what can be offered for these patients.

I have one plea. When we have a patient in front of us for a decision and that patient is blind or has some other problem, it is our policy to discuss it with the nursing staff, the technicians and the social worker to get a general opinion on what we think we can do. I have always been encouraged by the response of the supporting staff in the unit. They have always been very enthusiastic and they feel part of the decision-making process, and it is not just the nephrologist who makes the decision.

Cattell: I agree entirely that from the hard data we need more centres in Britain. I have no argument with Frank Parsons on this. We may disagree on how we get them. What does worry me, however, is the difficulties of recruiting nursing staff, certainly in the South-East of England, to the existing units. Before we rush headlong into setting up more units we should address ourselves yet again on how we can staff our existing units well.

I had hoped that Dr Gabriel would tell us how to get more nurses.

Gabriel: No.

V. Parsons: We have just discussed one of the problems which confronts dialysis units. In Dulwich Hospital, for the first time, we are to have learners, i.e. nurses in training, attached to the unit. Students will be coming to the unit and will see it. They should rotate throughout the unit. They should not do dialysis only but should go to the transplant wards and work there for a time and possibly help to run a transplant outpatient clinic. They should also see patients before they are in renal failure. It needs enormous flexibility on the part of the nursing administration to let nurses wander about, but if there are enough of them then it increases their interest, it enables them to do high-pressure stuff. This is very valuable and this is the way to offer a total exposure to nephrology and not just dialysis – which is where the hard work is done. All the other enjoyable things that keep nephrologists happy should be shared with the nursing staff. They should not just put needles in, take them out and keep the machines happy; they should also come to conferences like this.

F. M. Parsons: I should like to extend that. We made a howling error in the mid-1960s in the Working Party on the Establishment of Dialysis Units. This was really forced upon us. We built haemodialysis units in separate buildings so that inpatient care was done elsewhere.

If we are building new units then these must be integrated. The dialysis area must be alongside the inpatient renal area. This will give a variety of work for the staff.

We should not try to repeat the errors of the mid-1960's. Perhaps we should also tack on a transplant unit. The mixture of inpatient care and dialysis is vital when we come to a CAPD training programme and I hope that this will get through to the planners.

J. Walls (Leicester General Hospital): It seems that the gist of this morning's discussion is that we need more hospital-based haemodialysis facilities. Dr Pincherle has presented costings from three existing units in the UK. As haemodialysis by and large is currently home dialysis based, existing units are not necessarily run on the most economic lines for a hospital-based therapy.

We heard from Merseyside about the development of minimal care or satellite units. Has the DHSS looked at the costings for providing haemodialysis on a minimal care or satellite basis? Has it also looked at the costings in France, Italy, Germany or the United States, which now have very successful, large, hospital-based dialysis programmes, some of which are run on commercial lines where costing becomes of paramount importance? And what are the views on pursuing this line of therapy?

Pincherle: The DHSS originally found money for setting up six limited care units, one of them at Liverpool. I was slightly disappointed that no one mentioned that we had funded it. We also had funds to evaluate three of them including an economic evaluation. For a number of reasons the evaluation was slightly delayed and only started quite recently, but in a year or two's time we shall be able to have an economic evaluation comparing the costs in these limited care units with home dialysis and conventional hospital dialysis.

I entirely agree that limited care hospital dialysis should work out a lot cheaper than conventional hospital dialysis. We suspect that it may work out at not very much more than home dialysis.

We have not looked at costs in Germany, the USA and so on because there are so many differences that it is virtually impossible to make any meaningful comparisons. The salaries for staff, the costs of dialysis fluid, all these things are so different that it not worthwile making a comparison.

K. D. Nolph (University of Missouri): We all agree that there is great interest in using CAPD as a partial solution to the problem and that CAPD will indeed extend the facilities. But I hate the implication that facilities are being extended with a lesser form of therapy or that it is being bought mainly because it is cheaper.

The growth of CAPD in the United States has occurred against fiscal implications. Centre dialysis in our country has been reimbursed very very well, and for every patient that we place on centre haemodialysis we can make quite a profit. Every time we place a patient on CAPD we lose money. This may be changed in the near future but this has been so in the past, and, in spite of that, there are now over five hundred centres providing CAPD therapy. The reason is that they think that at least for some patients, CAPD is the best form of therapy that can be offered. Granted this is not so for all. But haemodialysis, if it is a gold standard, is tarnished for many patients. They develop symptoms and disequilibrium during dialysis. They feel poorly the day after and they have problems, sometimes significant complications, with blood access. There are life-threatening risks with haemodialysis. So it is certainly not a perfect therapy.

Neither is CAPD. CAPD also has its complications, and all of those who try CAPD may not succeed, and indeed they may need to go back to haemodialysis.

The best approach is to be able to offer all forms of therapy, and even change patients from one form of therapy to another as the need dictates.

There are indeed those who on haemodialysis have terrible problems. And in switching to CAPD they do very well. They have very little peritonitis. They feel much better all the time.

I have patients who on haemodialysis tell me they never felt well and now on CAPD they feel better every day. They tell me what it is like to stare at the wall and try and move the hands on the clock during haemodialysis therapy, and now on CAPD they are in control of their lives. This does not happen to everybody but it does happen to some, and for those it is a better form of therapy.

We are still in the phase of trial and error in trying to identify these patients, but I hate to hear the implication that a successful patient on CAPD is receiving a second rate therapy. I disagree.

Cattell: Were I to try to summarize this session I would say that Britain sadly lacks the facilities to provide this very successful form of renal replacement. Whether nephrologists are nice guys or nasty guys, we cannot get away from the fact that we have at this time underprovision of facilities.

Reference

Bone, J. M. (1978). Discussion, Section 3. In Anderton, J. L., Parsons, F. M. and Jones, D. E. (eds.). *Living with Renal Failure*. pp.99–100. (Lancaster: MTP Press)

SESSION TWO

An International Perspective
Chairman:
C. S. Ogg

Chairman's Introduction
C. S. Ogg

This morning, we had a splendid opening session which set the stage extremely well.

It seems to be quite obvious to people like myself, and more so to Dr Frank Parsons, that the name of the game has changed. We have spent the last 15 to 20 years exploring an exciting new form of medicine, showing that it worked, extending the indications. That exciting phase has gone and we are now in the position that we are convinced and have to sell our convictions to the world. We have almost to change our job from a medical one to a political one.

Our first three speakers this afternoon are all household names in dialysis and we are very fortunate to have three such eminent people with us. Our fourth speaker is someone whom I am looking forward to hearing even more than the others. This is because I believe very strongly that the solution to our current problem of the inability to match need to facilities, and our inability to deliver the goods, has to be a socio-economic one, and it has to come from government. Mr Carter-Jones, who will speak last, represents the All Party Group for the Disabled, from the Houses of Parliament.

I very much hope that either during the formal presentations or during discussion the speakers will take up Dr Parsons' challenge and also consider the legal aspects of our failure to treat people with treatable diseases. This has had quite a public airing within the past few months with the trial of Dr L. Arthur. During the course of that trial, counsel for the Crown suggested that the deliberate decision not to treat a patient having a treatable disease might justify a murder charge. In correspondence with one of the defence unions that point has been sustained, and if it really is true we shall be hearing a lot more from the lawyers. The day of reckoning may have come when we cease to get away with it.

All of us who are interested in CAPD are particularly grateful to the first speaker of the session, Professor Oreopoulos, for his work with the *Peritoneal Dialysis Bulletin*. I find it a very useful recipe book. I do not know how much science it contains but it is very nice to know what to do next. It appears regularly and updates us with the various new tricks that are available. I am looking forward to his talk.

6

Should we let them die?
D. G. Oreopoulos

6.1 INTRODUCTION

I would like to start by introducing four of my patients who are on treatment in our hospital's peritoneal dialysis unit. Mrs A. M. is a 91-year-old lady, an ex-professor of arts at the University of Toronto, who, on the days off dialysis, lives by herself in her home and is cared for by her neighbours. Mrs M. T. is a 65-year-old blind diabetic patient with both legs amputated,

who would not be accepted by any chronic care hospital; on her days off
dialysis she lives with one of her five daughters. Mrs H. is a 69-year-old
woman with systemic amyloidosis, bilateral hip arthritis requiring hip replacement, severe heart disease requiring a pacemaker and incapacitating
back pain. Finally, Mrs. K. is a 76-year-old patient with severe heart and
respiratory failure that prevents her from moving.

All these patients want to continue living on chronic intermittent peritoneal dialysis by coming twice a week to the hospital at a cost of approximately $160 000 per year. We could save $800 000 over the next five years if
we discontinued dialysis in these four patients and allowed them to die. In
this presentation I will try to discuss the moral, ethical and economic implications of this agonizing question.

6.2 BACKGROUND

The artificial kidney provided the first demonstration of effective organ replacement. The general adoption of maintenance dialysis has made professionals and many members of the public conscious of the impact that
artificial organ technology will have on our future, and has prepared the
way for a new specialty, a kind of 'spare part' medicine. This aspect of
medicine will soon be part of almost every specialty so that the complex
ethical, social and economic problems, which perplex the nephrologist
today, may become the problems of every specialist tomorrow. For this
reason, any lessons learned from our experience may help others avoid
difficulties or adapt to them in their own field in the future.

To understand these problems it may help if I review briefly, the development of the artificial kidney during the last three decades. The first artificial
kidney was developed by Dr W. Kolff in Holland during the Second World
War. In the 1950s, when only limited dialysis facilities were available around
the world, the treatment was reserved chiefly for patients with acute renal
failure, and for those with an exacerbation of chronic renal disease. Even
among these select patients, this extraordinary new procedure was provided
only to those who were very sick or terminally ill. Dialysis was performed
only by physicians, a new access to the vascular system had to be developed
each time, and the procedure, which took many hours, was often performed
during the night so that physicians could attend to their regular duties
during the day.

In the 1960s the development of Scribner's arteriovenous (AV) shunt
made chronic dialysis feasible for patients with end-stage renal disease
(ESRD). Society took a positive and favourable attitude to this life-support
treatment and was prepared to devote abundant resources to its application.
Technical developments solved many of the problems and dialysers were
produced in large numbers so that their scarcity was no longer a limiting
factor and theoretically all who needed treatment could have it. As a result,

although initially dialysis facilities were limited to those individuals who were judged to be valuable to society, facilities later seemed almost unlimited, and medical teams began to treat large numbers of patients including very old patients and those with additional chronic conditions such as diabetes, other systemic diseases and malignancies. Furthermore, social worthiness was no longer a criterion for treatment and nephrologists often offer dialysis to criminals and other individuals with deviant behaviour. In short, dialysis was changed from an extraordinary to an ordinary treatment.

6.3   THE ECONOMIC IMPLICATIONS

The principle that access to dialysis specifically and health care in general is the right of every individual has brought us face to face with a complex set of social, economic, political and ethical questions such as who should and should not be treated and whether treatment should be continued or discontinued. Questions about the quality of life, the right to die, and death with dignity are frequently raised and discussed in our daily rounds. Thus, while in the 1960s the big question about dialysis was, 'Why are we not providing abundant resources for this life-sustaining treatment?', the question in the 1980s has changed to, 'Why are we providing dialysis for everybody?'.

   This mix of socio-economic and moral problems is characteristic chiefly of the affluent and socially developed countries that can assign large proportions of their gross national products (GNP) to health care. There is a positive correlation between the number of dialysis patients per million of population in a country and the GNP of that country. In poor countries, treatment of diseases that respond to antibiotics, antiparasitic drugs or vaccines will save more lives than directing a limited health budget to the few patients dying from renal disease. An important difference between the costs incurred for dialysis patients and those with infectious diseases, is that the dialysis costs will continue year after year as long as the patients live. Furthermore, as long as the number of new patients entering the programme exceeds those leaving it (by death or transplantation), the total costs will continue to rise. The escalation of dialysis costs that took place in the USA between the years 1974 and 1979 took society by surprise and experience with the artificial kidney is now used as a warning of what may happen when research and technology make available other expensive artificial organs, such as the heart, pancreas and limbs. At the same time, various 'observers' regard the artificial kidney and other major technologies of today such as CAT scanners, coronary bypass surgery and electronic fetal monitoring as the major elements responsible for the increasing health care costs.

   Although most would agree that the remarkable advances in biomedical knowledge and developments in medical technology have helped to make modern medicine a substantial force for good in our world, a confrontation of increasing vigour is developing between those who would develop and apply medical technologies and those who must pay for them. The efforts of those who attack major medical technologies are made easier by the fact that we live in an era in which we are all aware of the disasters that technology has brought into our lives, such as environmental pollution and the threat of a nuclear war. As a result of these pressures the medical profession, even though it is composed of people trained to provide treatment, is now prepared to discuss whether a highly technological life support treatment, such as dialysis, should be rationed. We are being told that the goal of providing 'necessary' services to everyone 'without discrimination' belongs to the past and that because of the limitation of resources, certain people may have to be refused treatment.

6.4 MEDICAL RESPONSIBILITIES

What worries me is that, as physicians, we respond to these pressures by a process of rationalization in which we allow medical indications to be determined by economic considerations and thus, in some ways, we may be betraying the trust our patients have in us. Although future continuous financial restraints may change the rules that govern our relationship with our patients, we still attempt to follow the guidelines originally set down by Hippocrates, that the doctor should 'follow that system of regimen which, according to his ability and judgement, he considers the most beneficial for his patient'. Obviously Hippocrates had not even considered the possibility of withholding treatment (this is, in effect, what we are discussing today). His only concern was that the doctor should provide the best among those treatments available.

More recently, the World Medical Association adopted the rule that the ethical doctor must always bear in mind the obligation of preserving human life and that he owes his patient complete loyalty. Withholding a life support treatment would seem to go against this rule. Finally, and even more to the point, the Canadian Medical Association's Code of Ethics enjoins the ethical physician to first consider the well-being of the patient, and to recognize that the patient has the right to accept or reject any medical care recommended to him. If I was asked to revise this rule in any way, I would have added the word 'only' so that this rule would read, '*Only* the patient has the right to accept or reject a medical treatment'; nobody else can make this decision for him, assuming of course, that he or she is of sound mind. As long as society does not draw up explicit rules concerning the rationing of dialysis treatment (and as far as I know, none has done so), the only person who has the right to decide whether dialysis should be started and whether life with a machine is worth living, is the patient.

It should go without saying that the patient who faces the need for dialysis during the terminal stage of his renal disease should have placed clearly before him all the facts about the various treatments available. We now can offer seven or eight alternatives from which to choose a mode which best meets the individual patient's needs and the advantages and disadvantages of each of these should be made clear to the patient. He or she should also have an adequate description and full understanding of all the inconveniences and suffering that may arise if things do not turn out well and should be left alone to decide whether to continue living with a life support treatment. In my experience, everybody chooses to live. I would like to stress, however, that when dialysis is first considered, a uraemic patient may be confused and should be given the chance to make his own independent decision after the first few dialyses, when his mind has cleared.

To make my theme a little easier, I will take no position on the thorny issue of who has the right to decide whether dialysis should be started or continued in mentally incompetent patients. Recent court cases in the USA ended with conflicting decisions. Thus, whereas, in the Karen Ann Quinlan case the parents were granted the right to discontinue the life support treatment, in a more recent case the Court of Appeals decided that, 'minors and those who have never before expressed an opinion on their rights of dying, must undergo all treatments for a condition which threatens their life'. I should stress that, in most cases, we are confronted with the question of whether dialysis should be made available to mentally competent patients, like those I introduced at the beginning of this presentation. My own position is that, in Canada, and as long as a patient wants to live with dialysis, the treatment should be made available to him and nobody, not even his doctor, should have the right to pass judgement about the quality of his life and whether it is worth living. Recent history offers many examples of the terrible things that can happen once an individual or a group of individuals gain the right to make decisions about the worth of another's life.

Once a treatment has been started, it is morally wrong to discontinue it for financial reasons. Even in the early years of dialysis, when we were practising patient selection, patients had the full support of the team, once they had been accepted into the programme. On the other hand, the patient who has decided to start treatment, should be provided with a guarantee that if things did not go well, and he wished to discontinue treatment he could do so at any time. From time to time, we should remind the patients of their rights in this respect.

I would go even further and say that when the patient is agonizing over the decision of whether or not to continue on the life-support treatment, we should make available to him professionals such as the hospital's chaplain, the psychiatrist and the social worker who may help him to decide. Of course, doctors and nurses should be at ease when they discuss with their patients the option of death.

6.5 THE IMPOSITION OF RESTRICTIONS

With few exceptions, I think that both the Ministry of Health and the individual hospital boards will avoid explicit rationing of dialysis services such as that conveyed in a letter I received from two, well known chronic care hospitals which bluntly stated that dialysis patients will not be accepted. These explicit restrictions will become increasingly common as we become, to a greater and greater extent, a society of isolated individuals with less and less compassion for those who suffer. In the meantime, most of the restrictions will continue to be implicit, such as are inherent in fixed budgets, which are part of the global budget of the hospital and in restrictions on the sites of care, in the number of hospital beds, and in the number of specialty positions. By restricting the budget and insisting that the dialysis budget should be included in the hospital's global budget, health administrators are creating a situation in which one of two things may happen, depending on the strength and aggressiveness of the nephrology department. Either the dialysis programme will continue to provide its services to everybody at the expense of other departments; or, if the nephrologists are not sufficiently aggressive or become fed-up with the situation, services will be provided only to selected patients and the remainder will have to look for other hospitals or die. In the latter case, I fear that nephrologists, *instead* of telling the patients the real reasons behind this inability to provide treatment, will abuse their trust and cover up the government's economic restraints by propounding plausible 'medical' reasons why the treatment should not or could not be started.

Implicit restrictions are as effective as explicit ones, and avoid the embarrassment of specifying the type of services that should be restricted, thus allowing those who govern us to avoid reaction and confrontation. They achieve their goals by placing greater pressure on the medical staff to make difficult allocation decisions.

6.6 THE MEDICAL RESPONSE

I believe that the medical profession should be prepared to take up the challenge of making the difficult decisions which result from the implicit restrictions, under the following terms:

(a) We should accept responsibility for choices between waste and saving but not between life and death.

(b) The public should be made fully aware of the process so that, in its confusion, it will not blame the profession for the resulting limitations.

The first challenge is that of controlling health care costs. In most countries, these are between 8 and 9% of the GNP and compete with other major areas of expenditure such as defence, energy, education and crime control.

Even though I do not accept that in order to increase defence expenditure we have to undermine the support of an excellent health care system, I am afraid that the forces opposing the expansion of the health sector are so strong that, at present, we may as well accept this as a fact.

In trying to find ways of achieving economy without jeopardizing quality, a difficult, if not impossible, task in many cases, we must look at the reasons for recent increases in health-care costs. Advanced technology is only one of these, so that an attack on technology alone will not bring the desired economies. Instead we should direct our efforts to the development of a mix of techniques, which are responsive to the patient's needs, and at the same time allow the physician to exercise discretion and clinical judgement whilst protecting the public purse.

We can achieve significant savings if we teach ourselves and each new generation of medical students and doctors to *think* instead of relying on 'routine' investigations to provide the diagnosis. Recently I heard Dr S. Lenkie, a colleague of mine, saying to her residents, 'Thinking is painful but very profitable'. We must bring about fundamental changes in the values which physicians develop during their medical education. We must make a shift towards a value system that rewards the discriminating use of selected diagnostic and therapeutic procedures. We also need a system that rewards cost-efficient providers and provides financial incentives, which encourage efficiency and reduce waste. In the field of dialysis we can achieve this by promoting home or self-care dialysis. In home or self-care dialysis the patient takes over some of the responsibility of his care and, in return, regains his independence. Of course, not all patients will accept this treatment so it is up to us to promote its advantages. Although some patients resent it, I see no problem in explaining that they have to share some of the burden of their own treatment if dialysis is to become available to everybody. Significant savings can be achieved by re-use of dialysers. If properly done, this causes only a minor degree of morbidity and should be acceptable to both patients and doctors. Savings may also be achieved by the centralization of certain services and the avoidance of duplication of services. Such a move may demand personal sacrifices from doctors already established but, in this era of financial restraints, duplication often results in a significant waste.

Finally, for suitable patients, the promotion of transplantation can contribute to a significant saving. I believe that Canadian nephrologists have done their part since, in Canada, we treat almost as many patients with ESRD as in any country without having, at our disposal, expensive private dialysis facilities. We have been able to do this by promoting home dialysis, self-care dialysis and transplantation – all of which, represent important economies. However, the increasing number of patients on home dialysis and transplantation imposes a heavy burden on expensive in hospital dialysis facilities because whenever these treatments fail, the patients need back-up hospitalization. Furthermore, the liberalization of our admission criteria and the acceptance of old patients and those with other systemic diseases, creates a demand for extra nursing, even when the number of patients does not increase substantially.

6.7 POLITICAL RESPONSIBILITY

If politicians insist on restraining health care costs, they should take the responsibility of telling the public that under these circumstances their expectations of superior medical care for every citizen cannot be fulfilled. After all, politicians usually are ready to respond to the wishes of the public and we, as providers of health care, cannot meet two opposing requests, namely to reduce costs and to provide excellent services to all patients. While doctors have the responsibility to do their best without waste, it is up to the public and their elected representatives to develop a philosophy to justify choices, which are becoming increasingly complex, and to decide what place health care should be assigned in their list of priorities. The nephrologists, the entire medical profession, industry, the public and government must move beyond prejudice and mistrust and cooperate in searching for a solution, so that our future priorities and the final place of health care may be established.

I am sure that as long as there is trust between doctors, government and patients, the costs of a life-support treatment such as dialysis, can be handled effectively and, at the same time, this service will be made available to all who need it.

6.8 RECOMMENDATIONS

Specifically, I would suggest that:

(A) The Ministry of Health should handle the dialysis budget under a separate programme and outside the hospitals' global budget.

(B) Nephrologists should demonstrate to the public and to the government that their fight for more and better services is the result of a genuine interest in their patients' welfare and is not motivated by a desire to make more money and to build larger 'empires'.

(C) Patients should band together so as to use the lobbying power of their associations to convince the government to provide the necessary funding to meet the needs of patients with ESRD. The Kidney Foundation, both local and national, should include in their goals, the application of pressure on the government for an increase in health support. As their advisors, we have a special role to play and have a special responsibility to describe the problem clearly.

A public that has been sold the concept that superior health care is a right of every citizen must realize that, unless health care is accorded a higher priority at present, that right will be steadily eroded.

(D) We should press society and government to take a stand and declare whether or not expensive life-support treatments should be provided to everyone. Up to now, the government has not faced up to the issue and by applying implicit restrictions has hoped to force doctors to decide who should live and who should die.

6.9 CONCLUSION

In this presentation I have tried to highlight a series of problems that will increasingly affect the medical profession within the next decade or two. I am sure that the profession will respond to the challenge that is imposed by the financial restraints of our times and will do its best to save money by avoiding waste. However, I think that, under no circumstances, should we compromise and betray the trust that our patients have in us, by agreeing to consider rationing any life-support treatment for the sake of economy.

References for future reading

Following is a list of some of the references that I think should be read by those who are interested in this topic. My apologies to all other authors whose articles I have read before preparing this article and who are not mentioned individually. I will be happy to provide these references on request.

Friedman, E. A. and Delano, B. G. (1981). Can the world afford uremia therapy? In Zurukzoglu, W. M., Papadimitriou, M., Pyrpasopoulos, M., Sion, C. and Zamboulis, C. (eds.) *Proceedings 8th International Congress of Nephrology,* pp. 577–583 (Basel: Karger)

Galetti, P. M. (1979). Organ replacement technology: its impact on the quality and cost of medical care. Frank W. Hastings lecture. NIH contractors meeting, Devices and Technology Branch, December 10–12

Parsons, V. (1978). The ethical challenges of dialysis and transplantation. *Practitioner,* **220,** 871

Parsons, V. and Lock, P. (1980). Triage and the patient with renal failure. *J. Med. Ethics,* **6,** 173

Fox, C. (1981). Exclusion from dialysis: a sociologic and legal perspective. *Kidney Int.,* **19,** 739

7

Dialysis and transplantation in the United States and the impact of continuous ambulatory peritoneal dialysis (CAPD)
K. D. Nolph

7.1 INTRODUCTION

In 1972, the Social Security Act was amended to authorize funding for the
treatment of end-stage renal disease under Medicare. At that time about 40
patients per million population were receiving longterm haemodialysis
treatment and 40% of dialysis treatments were home-based (Relman, 1980).
Now, a decade later, patients on dialysis treatment in the United States
exceed 250 per million population. Less than 15% are dialysed at home
(*End-stage Renal Disease*, 1980; *Quarterly Statistical Summary*, 1981; *The
Kidney Dialysis Industry*, 1981).

Continuous ambulatory peritoneal dialysis (CAPD) is a newer alternative
form of home dialysis (Nolph, 1981a). It was first offered in Texas in 1975.
As of January 1982, over 5000 patients were being treated in the US with
this form of therapy (*The Kidney Dialysis Industry*, 1981). New proposed
Medicare reimbursement regulations offer incentives for all types of home
dialysis (Iglehart, 1982). These fiscal incentives coupled with other
attractive characteristics of CAPD are expected to increase its use (*The
Kidney Dialysis Industry*, 1981).

It is the purpose of this paper to provide an overview of dialysis and
transplant activities in the United States, to review the impact of CAPD to
date and to give some predictions as to the role of CAPD in the future.

7.2 EXTENT AND DISTRIBUTION OF THERAPY FOR END-STAGE RENAL DISEASE IN THE US

We will define end-stage renal disease (ESRD) as renal failure to the degree
that uraemic symptoms become incapacitating without intervention by
dialysis or transplant (*End-stage Renal Disease*, 1981). In 1980, the Health
Care Finance Administration submitted their second annual report to Congress on ESRD (Relman, 1980). This report covered the full range of
activities related to the care of ESRD patients in 1979. At the end of that
year there were 45 565 patients on chronic dialysis, a 25% increase over the
previous year. The home dialysis population consisted of 5941 patients
(13%). During that year, 4271 kidney transplants were performed, 1205 were
from living-related donors (28.2%) and the rest were from cadaver donors.

Some of this data was updated by the Health Care Finance Administration in late 1981. As of 31 December 1980 there were 61 443 patients entitled
to Medicare payments for ESRD therapy (see Table 7.1). Payments for
therapy during 1980 totalled $1 207 600 000. As of 7 July 1981, there were
156 transplant centres and 1093 dialysis facilities or centres approved for reimbursement. As of 12 January 1981 536 haemodialysis home training
centres and 381 CAPD training centres had been approved. 4697 kidney
transplants were performed in 1980. As of 31 December 1980 9% of the
patients were on home haemodialysis and 4.5% were on CAPD.

Table 7.1   US Medicare

No. of patients	61 443	(1980)
Payments	$1 207 600 000	(1980)
Transplant centres	156	(7 July 1981)
Dialysis facilities and centres	1 093	(7 July 1981)
Haemodialysis home training centres	536	(12 January 1981)
CAPD training centres	382	(12 January 1981)
Kidney transplants	4 697	(1980)

(from *End-Stage Renal Disease*, 1980)

7.3   COMPARATIVE ANNUAL COSTS

The Bernstein Research Institute has estimated comparative costs of different forms of therapy in the US during 1981 (see Table 7.2) (*The Kidney Dialysis Industry*, 1981). Annual costs were calculated over five years for many categories and include training fees, physicians' fees, surgical procedures, equipment costs, annual supply costs and average hospitalization costs. The reader is referred to the references for more details. Clearly, however, home dialysis techniques and successful kidney transplantation are of potentially lower cost than centre haemodialysis when calculated on an annual basis.

Table 7.2   Comparative annual costs (1981)

Haemodialysis	
hospital	$28 800
centre	$24 100
home	$14 850
Peritoneal Dialysis .	
reverse osmosis	$19 000
cycler	$21 000
CAPD	$18 300
CCPD	$19 700
Transplant	$10 000

(from *The Kidney Dialysis Industry*, 1981)

Table 7.3   US Medicare transplantation costs and charges

Average kidney acquisition charge (1981)	
living related	$7 581
cadaveric	$6 992
Average charge/transplant	$20 156
Estimated cost/transplant	$14 403

(from *End-Stage Renal Disease*, 1980)

Table 7.3 summarizes figures relative to kidney transplantation costs and changes released by the Health Care Finance Administration (*End-stage Renal Disease*, 1980; *Quarterly Statistical Summary*, 1981). Average kidney acquisition charges, average charge per transplant and estimated cost per transplant are shown. Transplantation costs are relatively high during the immediate transplant period, but the annual costs of a successful kidney transplant fall well below those of dialysis therapy.

7.4 CHRONIC DIALYSIS BY TYPE OF SETTING

Table 7.4 shows a breakdown of the distribution of chronic dialysis by the type of setting (1980) based on Bernstein figures. Centre dialysis was dominant. Free-standing centres (independent of a hospital) were mainly of the non-profit type.

Table 7.4   Chronic dialysis by type of setting (1980)

Hospitals	47.1%
Free standing centres	
for profit	30.8%
non-profit	7.7%
Home care	14.4%
	100.0%

(from *End-stage Renal Disease*, 1980)

7.5 SURVIVAL RATES

Table 7.5 shows one-year survival rates for males in different age groups regardless of the type of ESRD therapy. Results during a period in the early 1970s are compared to results obtained four years later. Based on this national data from the Health Care Finance Administration, there has been no significant change in patient survival (*End-stage Renal Disease*, 1980). The probability of death for the ESRD population is more than 50–100

Table 7.5   One year survival rates (males) (combined dialysis and transplantation)

Age	Oct 1973–Sept 1974	Oct 1977–Sept 1978
5–14	0.888	0.979
15–24	0.910	0.913
25–34	0.891	0.881
35–44	0.837	0.858
45–54	0.833	0.828
55–64	0.805	0.774
65–74	0.686	0.704
75 +	0.579	0.594

(from *End-Stage Renal Disease*, 1980)

times the probability for the US population for the younger age groups. The difference in death rates between ESRD patients and normals decreases with increasing age, but is still 5–15 times above normal for ESRD patients in the over-65 population. Each cohort is composed of individuals whose date of entry into the ESRD programme is within the year long period indicated. The survival rate for each cohort group is the proportion of people still living one year after the entry date.

There are additional data on patient survival from different regions in the United States. A recent report analysing survival of ESRD patients in the state of Michigan shows survival data in more than 2000 ESRD patients from 1974 through 1978 (Weller *et al.*, 1982). Five year survival for home haemodialysis patients was 50% compared with 32% for centre haemodialysis ($p = 0.01$). Survival after transplantation from a related donor was 75% at five years, and was also significantly higher than the survival of centre dialysis patients ($p = 0.01$). Patient survival following transplantation from cadaver donors and the survival of haemodialysis patients were nearly identical at five years. It must be kept in mind that such differences largely reflect patient selection practices and do not represent age-matched randomized comparisons of different therapies. Nevertheless, these figures do reflect what has been happening in the State of Michigan.

Table 7.6 Dialysis and transplantation rates per 100 000 population in Missouri (1 July 1980–30 June 1981)

Chronic dialysis*	
white	14.21
non-white	56.19
total	19.09
Transplantation	
white	6.83
non-white	12.25
total	7.44

*(as of 30 June 1981) (from *Missouri Kidney Program*, 1980)

7.6 EXPERIENCES IN THE STATE OF MISSOURI

Another region which has been monitoring ESRD therapy is the state of Missouri. The Missouri Kidney Program sponsored by the state maintains an extensive system for monitoring ESRD activities in Missouri. Table 7.6 summarizes dialysis and transplantation activities in Missouri between 1 July 1980 and 30 June 1981 (*Missouri Kidney Program*, 1982). The number of patients on chronic dialysis per 100 000 population is much higher in the non-whites. The number of kidney transplants performed per year per 100 000 population also seems to be much higher in the non-white population. This agrees with numerous observations suggesting a higher incidence of ESRD in the black population. Table 7.7 shows the high pro-

Table 7.7   Racial distribution of populations in Missouri

	% non-whites
Total Missouri population	11.6%
Dialysis population	34.2%
Transplant population	19.1%

(from *Missouri Kidney Program*, 1980)

portion of non-whites receiving various ESRD therapies. Whereas non-whites represent 11.6% of the total Missouri population, they represent 34.2% of the dialysis population and 19.1% of the transplant population.

Table 7.8   Dialysis deaths in Missouri

	%
Myocardial infarction	14.8
Pericarditis	2.1
Cardiac (other)	29.6
Cerebrovascular	2.7
Haemorrhage	3.2
Infection	6.3
Malignancy	1.6

(from *Missouri Kidney Program*, 1980)

Table 7.8 summarizes the causes of dialysis deaths in the State of Missouri from 1 July 1980 to 30 June 1981. Cardiovascular causes of death predominate. Small percentages of deaths are due to haemorrhage, usually gastrointestinal, infections and malignancies. All other causes of death account for very small percentages and are not shown.

Table 7.9   Cumulative survival of patients in Missouri

	1	2	3	4	5	
Patients on chronic dialysis	0.84	0.73	0.65	0.58	0.51	(*n* = 861)
Patients transplanted at least once	0.94	0.89	0.85	0.81	0.79	(*n* = 1735)
Living related graft survival	0.80	0.80	–	–	–	(*n* = 95)
Cadaveric graft survival	0.44	0.39	0.33	0.32	0.30	(*n* = 471)

(from *Missouri Kidney Program*, 1980)

Table 7.9 summarizes the cumulative survival of patients receiving different treatments in the State of Missouri, using data obtained since the programme began over ten years ago. Patients on chronic dialysis appear to have lower survivals than those transplanted at least once. This again reflects the selection of younger and healthier patients for transplant programmes. Graft survival figures are also shown for recipients of living-related and cadaver transplants. One year survival in the former is 80% while in the latter it is 44%.

Analyses of patient survival with different techniques in the State of Missouri over different time periods suggest improved survival figures for younger (20–39 years) chronic dialysis patients and living-related transplant patients in recent years, as compared to earlier experiences (Rikli *et al.*, in press).

Table 7.10 Reimbursement sources in Missouri (1980–81) (figures in US $)

Total charges (25 centres)	26 344 787
Payments	
Medicare (federal)	16 673 514
Medicaid (state)	1 028 791
Missouri Kidney Program (state)	1 323 175
other	4 186 126
Unpaid	3 033 081

(from *Missouri Kidney Program*, 1980)

Table 7.10 shows a breakdown of who pays for ESRD therapy in the state of Missouri (*Missouri Kidney Program*, 1980) as reflected by data collected during the fiscal year from mid-1980 to mid-1981. Total charges rendered by 25 centres were $26 344 787 00. Medicare paid 63% of these charges, Medicaid 4% and the Missouri Kidney Program 5%. Other payees, such as insurance companies, paid 16%. This left about 12% unpaid and presumably covered by institutional or supplier resources.

Figure 7.1 shows a detailed analysis of the epidemiology of ESRD in Missouri from 1 July 1980 to 30 June 1981. These figures are developed from multiple sources and, in some cases, must include estimates. However, this complicated diagram gives some indication as to the incidence of kidney disease in the total population and the numbers of patients with kidney disease who go on to ESRD. The flow of patients from different forms of therapy can be appreciated.

Table 7.11 USA Chronic dialysis population

	1980	1982(E)	1984(E)
Haemodialysis	52 500	56 695	58 350
Peritoneal dialysis	2 475	7 275	11 550
Total	54 975	63 970	69 900

(E) = estimated average for year
(from *The Kidney Dialysis Industry*, 1981)

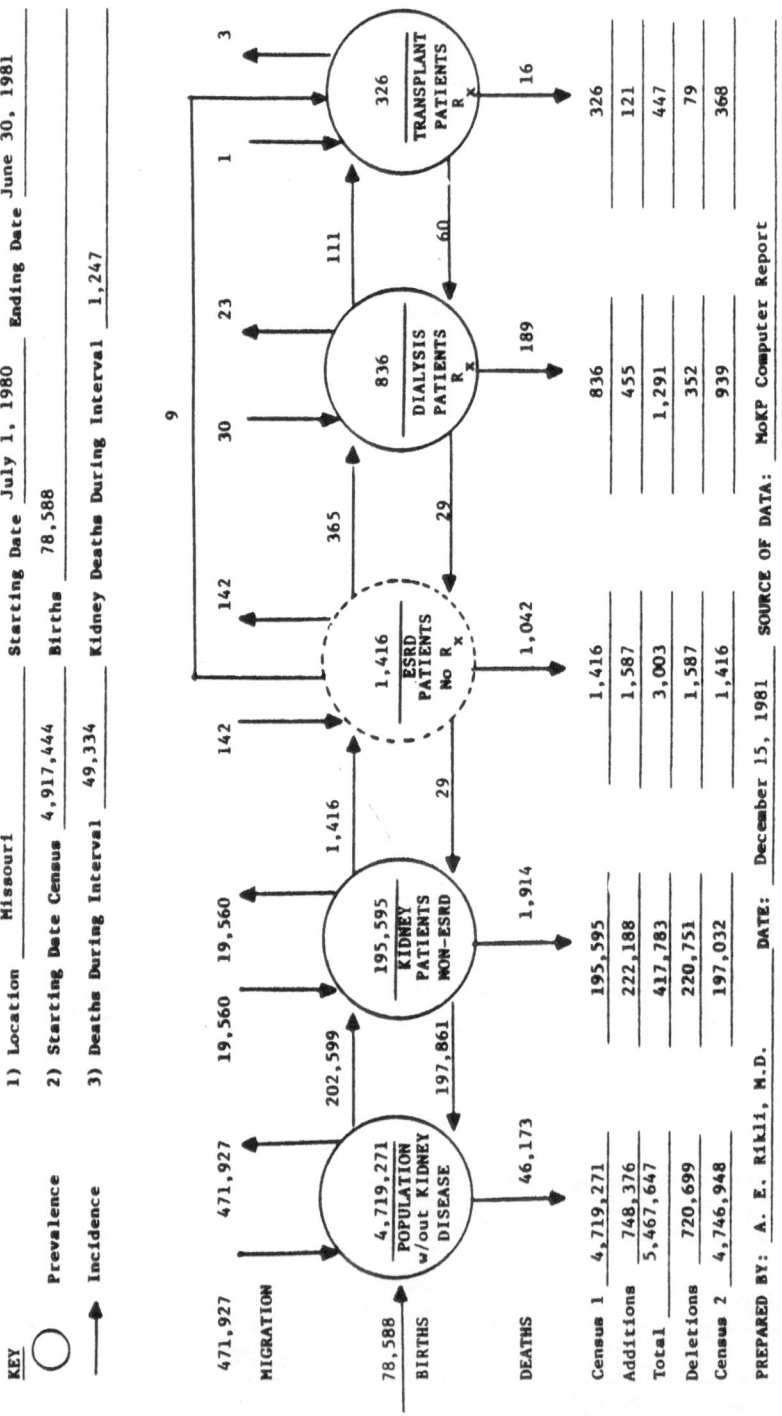

Figure 7.1 Missouri Kidney Program epidemiology of end-stage renal disease

Table 7.12   New patient entry rate

	Rate/million	Total
1980	76.0	17 214
1984(E)	77.4	18 228

(E) = estimated average for year
(from *The Kidney Dialysis Industry*, 1981)

7.7   PROJECTIONS

The Bernstein Research Institute has made interesting projections about expected changes in the ESRD population in coming years (*The Kidney Dialysis Industry*, 1981). Table 7.11 shows the US chronic dialysis population in 1980 (according to Bernstein figures) and estimated figures for 1982 and 1984. The proportionately greater growth in the number of patients receiving peritoneal dialysis reflects the anticipated increase in CAPD. Table 7.12 shows projected patient entry rates based on 1980 data and estimates for 1984. These new patients will add to the ESRD population as shown in Table 7.13 and coupled with returns from failed transplants and minus new successful transplants, will result in net new patients as indicated. The net growth in the dialysis population, however, will be less than this due to deaths of patients on chronic dialysis. Based on predicted mortalities in 1984 and observed mortalities in 1980, the actual net growth in the chronic dialysis population is indicated at the bottom of Table 7.13. We will thus be approaching between 250 and 300 chronic dialysis patients per million population.

Table 7.13   USA dialysis population forecast

	New patients		Returns from transplant		New transplants		Net new patients
1980	17 214	+	1 069	–	4 583	=	13 700*
1984(E)	18 228	+	1 278	–	5 517	=	13 989**

*1980 net increase from 52 262 to 57 688
**1984 net increase from 68 862 to 71 038
(E) Estimated average for year
(from *The Kidney Dialysis Industry*, 1981)

The average size of the home dialysis population in 1980 and that expected in 1984 are shown in Table 7.14. Home haemodialysis is projected to decrease, CAPD to increase remarkably (it is already over the 5000 mark) and home intermittent peritoneal dialysis (IPD) is projected to decrease while continuous cyclic peritoneal dialysis (CCPD) will also increase. Largely because of the increase in CAPD and CCPD, the total home population will increase from 14.4 to 22.2% of the dialysis population.

Table 7.14   Average home dialysis population

	1980	1984(E)
Haemodialysis	5725	4200
CAPD	1510	9650
IPD	650	200
CCPD	15	1500
Total	7900	15500
As % of total dialysis population	14.4%	22.2%

(from *The Kidney Dialysis Industry*, 1981)

Table 7.15   Average patients on CAPD

	Number	% of dialysis population
1980	1 500	2.7
1982(E)	5 925	9.3
1985(E)	11 200	15.6

(E) Estimate average for year
(from *The Kidney Dialysis Industry*, 1981)

Table 7.15 summarizes the numbers of patients on CAPD in 1980 and the projections for 1982 and 1985. Thus, in 1985, it is anticipated that 15.6% of the US dialysis population will be on CAPD.

7.8   THE NATIONAL CAPD REGISTRY

The National Institute of Health is sponsoring a CAPD registry (Nolph, 1981b). Over 3000 patients on CAPD are being monitored and the registry is attempting to monitor all US CAPD patients. Follow-up data has been analysed from 13 centres during the first nine months of 1981 when 481 patients began or entered CAPD programmes at these centres. Table 7.16

Table 7.16   13 Centre pilot study (1 January 1981–30 September 1981), last reported status

Status	No. of patients	%
CAPD	378	78.4
Haemodialysis	47	9.8
Died	30	6.2
IPD	11	2.3
Transplant	9	1.9
Return of renal function	5	1.0
Lost to follow-up	2	0.4
	482	100.0

shows the last reported status of these patients. 78% remained on CAPD after nine months. Table 7.17 shows the months on dialysis, months on CAPD, and days under observation during this nine month period. Mean, minimum, and maximum values are shown. A number of patients have been transferred from other forms of dialysis therapy so that the average number of months on chronic dialysis exceeds the months on CAPD. Note that the longest a patient has been maintained on CAPD is 52 months.

Table 7.17   13 Centre pilot study (1 January 1981 – 30 September 1981)

	Mean	*Min.*	*Max.*
Months on dialysis	29.3	0.03	192
Months on CAPD	12.7	0.03	52
Days on study	172	1.0	273

Table 7.18   Diabetic status, 13 centre pilot study (1 January 1981 – 30 September 1981)

Non-diabetic	76%
Diabetic	
intraperitoneal insulin	14.3%
subcutaneous insulin	3.7%
no insulin	3.5%
subcutaneous and	
intraperitoneal insulin	1.7%

Table 7.18 shows the distribution of CAPD patients in these 13 centres relative to their diabetic status. 24% of all patients are considered diabetics and 14.3% of all patients received intraperitoneal insulin.

Table 7.19 shows the annual rates for selected outcome measures in these 482 CAPD patients followed for 226.75 patient years. Survival data and actuarial analyses of these outcome measures will be developed as the data base increases. In our programme, the 2 year patient survival on CAPD is 85% and the technique success with solutions in plastic bags is 63% at 2 years.

Table 7.19   Annual rates for selected occurrences computed from data on 482 CAPD patients followed for 226.75 patient-years at 13 centres

Occurrence	*Patients having one or more occurrence*	*Occurrences patient/year*
Peritonitis episodes	234	2.07
Exit site/tunnel infections	112	0.79
Catheter replacements	76	0.40
Hospital admissions	297	2.73
Days hospitalized (any person)	313	27.09
Days trained	217	8.43

7.9 COMMENTS

It can be seen that, in the United States, the availability of federal funds for ESRD therapy was associated with a shift in therapy toward centre dialysis. Part of this can be explained by the fact that reimbursement policies provided fiscal disincentives for home dialysis. Anticipated changes in reimbursement policies may cause a shift once again in the direction of home therapy. Good comparisons of cumulative survival using home versus centre therapy are not available. Surveys and registries primarily focus on patient selection policies rather than direct comparisons of techniques. Thus, trends away from and now possibly toward home therapy may reflect fiscal matters rather than differences in medical outcomes.

CAPD has many attractions as a dialysis technique per se. It is internal, potentially less expensive, provides steady chemical control, does not require blood access, does not require a machine, requires a short training period, and offers self therapy. The growth of CAPD began without fiscal incentives and, in fact, in the presence of fiscal disincentives. Thus, changes to reimburse CAPD more fairly may stimulate even more growth than in the past and in current projections.

CAPD is not without problems. Peritonitis continues to be a recurring problem in many patients and explains the relatively high dropout rates from this technique. Dextrose absorption from the peritoneal cavity can contribute to obesity and to hyperlipidaemia. New connectors and new osmotic agents may solve both of these problems. Thus, future developments which affect the rates of complications of CAPD may also have tremendous impact on eventual growth rates.

Thus, CAPD is undergoing a rapid rate of growth which is projected to continue. The growth of CAPD will have a significant influence on the distribution of the chronic dialysis patients between home and centre dialysis therapy.

References

End-Stage Renal Disease: Pathophysiology, Dialysis and Transplantation. (1981). National Center for Health Care Technology, Monograph Series. US Department of Health and Human Services

End-Stage Renal Disease, Second Annual Report to Congress, FY 1980, by Department of Health and Human Services, Health Care Financing Administration, Baltimore, MD (1981)

Iglehart, J. K. (1982). Funding the end-stage renal disease program. *N. Engl. J. Med.,* **306,** 492

Missouri Kidney Program Annual Report. July 1, 1980 to June 30, 1981. (1982). Rikli, E., Coordinator, University of Missouri-Columbia, Columbia, MO 65201.

Nolph, K. D. (1981a). Continuous ambulatory peritoneal dialysis, Editorial Review, *Am. J. Nephrol.,* **1,** 1

Nolph, K. D. (1981b). Principal investigator, the National Registry pilot study group: the National Registry of CAPD patients. *Dial. Transpl.,* **10,** 744

Quarterly Statistical Summary (1981). By the Office of End-Stage Renal Disease, Health Care Financing Administration, Office of Special Programs, Baltimore, MD

Relman, A. S. (1980). The New Medical-Industrial Complex. *N. Engl. J. Med.,* **303,** 963

Rikli, A. E., Kappel, D. F. and Austin, D. (1982). Change in survival of ESRD patients treated during the past 15 years. (in press)

The Kidney Dialysis Industry, Bernstein Research (1981). C. Bernstein & Co., Inc., Member, New York Stock Exchange, New York, NY

Weller, J. M., Port, F. K., Swartz, R. D., Ferguson, C. W., Williams, G. W. and Jacobs, J. F. (1982). Analysis of survival of end-stage renal disease patients. *Kidney Int.,* **21,** 78

8

Treating end-stage renal failure in Italy
G. d'Amico

8.1 INTRODUCTION

We have available in Italy a national registry of all dialysis and transplant patients which is run by the 'Associazione Nazionale Emodializzati' (ANED), the Italian association of dialysis patients. It is a very useful source of information for all surveys in this field in our country; the data are more complete than those of the EDTA registry and are very accurate, because of the direct control of the individual patient data in every single facility.

8.2   DIALYSIS

I will refer to the ANED data in this chapter. Figures 8.1 and 8.2 show the progressive growth in the number of dialysis facilities and patients from 1972 to 1980 in Italy. When allowance is made for deaths and successful transplantation, it can be calculated that 35 new patients per million of population per year entered the regular dialysis (RDT) programme in 1972, and that this figure rose to over 55 per million per year during 1980. This is quite different from the figure of 34.2 per million population reported by the EDTA registry (Jacobs *et al.,* 1981). In fact, 3174 new patients started

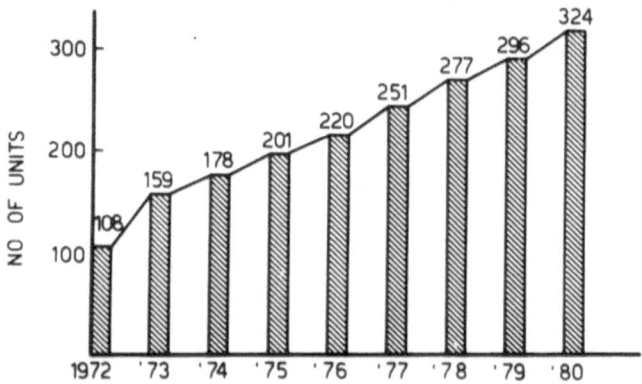

Figure 8.1   Total number of public and private dialysis units in Italy during the years 1972–1980

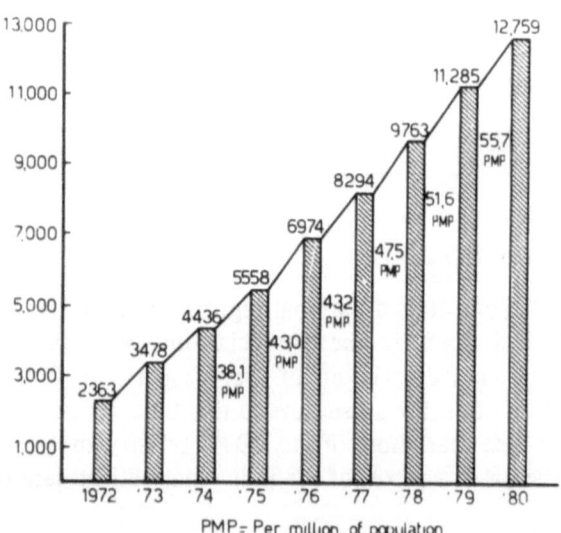

PMP = Per million of population

Figure 8.2   Total number of patients on regular dialysis treatment in Italy during the years 1972–1980

RDT in 1980 instead of the 1937 reported by the EDTA registry. The definitive data are not yet available for 1981, but preliminary results show that the total number of patients on RDT at the end of 1981 exceeds 14 000, and suggest that more than 50 new patients per million population started RDT during the year.

Table 8.1 Patients per million of population on regular dialysis treatment at 31 December 1980 in some European countries (EDTA registry) and in Italy (ANED registry)

Switzerland	259.7
Belgium	233.1
France	228.6
Italy	223.8
Fed. Rep. of Germany	208.0

As Table 8.1 shows, using the more complete data of the ANED survey, Italy had the fourth highest number of uraemic patients receiving RDT per million population in Europe at the end of 1980. However, the achievement of such high figures in our country has been accompanied by a great waste of money, due to the inefficient use of existing facilities, lack of co-ordinated planning and inadequate management by both national and regional health administrators.

8.2.1 Finance and facilities available

Dialysis patients in Italy are legally entitled to free treatment. There is no regionally imposed policy to limit the financial provision and this has favoured the growth of dialysis facilities, since regional and hospital administrators are being virtually 'blackmailed' by the arrival of each new patient at the terminal life-threatening stage of uraemia. The dramatic ultimatum of the nephrologist cannot be evaded easily.

The reimbursement policy, whereby a fixed fee is given to physicians running private dialysis facilities for in-centre dialysis, has favoured the proliferation of such facilities, as it did in the USA (Blagg and Scribner, 1980). This is especially true in central and southern Italy, where hospital facilities in general have always been scarce and deficient and each new publicly financed unit is harder to organize than its predecessors.

The analysis of the distribution of patients among the different modalities of dialysis treatment, shown for the whole country and for some sample Regions in Table 8.2 requires some comment.

(1) The total number of public and private dialysis units is very large. From the national average of 40 patients per unit, it is obvious that the majority cater for too few patients.

Table 8.2 Number of centres and patients on regular dialysis treatment (RDT) in Italy at the end of 1980

	Total population (millions)	No. of dialysis units			Total no. of patients on RDT				patient deaths during 1980 (%)
		public hospital units	private facilities	public limited care centres	per million population	on home haemodialysis (%)	on CAPD or IPD (%)	on limited care (%)	
Italy	57.0	247	77	78	223.8	7.7	3.2	6.7	9.3
Lombardia	8.9	30	5	22	258	22.6	4.8	10.7	5.4
Piemonte	4.6	19	–	10	255	15.7	2.7	14.4	9.2
Lazio	5.0	19	17	–	182	0.6	0	0	14.4
Sicilia	5.0	20	23	–	227	0.2	0.2	0	11.8
Sardegna	1.6	9	1	–	170	3.3	3.3	0	9.4

(2) This situation is a consequence of the insufficient development of self-care dialysis, and in particular of home dialysis, mainly in the private profit-making institutions, but also in the hospital units. In the private establishments there is a definite financial advantage to physicians in continuing in-centre treatment; the alternative home treatment requires by regional law several troublesome and expensive extensions of the available facilities such as 24-hour staffing, the availability of machines for hospital back-up, etc. In publicly financed hospitals there is no incentive to start home dialysis programmes, with the consequent increase in work and responsibility. Special laws regulate home and limited care dialysis in almost every region, but there has not been sufficient pressure exerted on physicians in the public sector to increase home dialysis, as the cheaper treatment allowing better rehabilitation. Thus in large areas of Italy, no effort has been made to reduce the prejudice of many patients against self-care and their dependence on the hospital environment, prejudice that is used as an 'alibi' by physicians and administrators.

(3) The great variation in the policies carried out in the different regions explains the substantial differences in the type and quality of the treatment provided to local populations. At the end of 1980 in Lombardia, the region of northern Italy where Milan is situated, 35 units, nearly all situated in public hospitals, provided RDT to 2310 patients (258 per million population), 27.4% of whom were being treated at home and 10.7% in limited care centres, with an overall mortality of 5.4% in 1980 (Table 8.2). At the same time, in Lazio, the region in central Italy where Rome is situated, in a comparable number of units (36), the majority of which were private profit-making institutions, less than half the number of patients (921 *vs.* 2310) were being treated. Only 0.6% of these were at home or in limited care centres, with an overall mortality in 1980 nearly three times higher than in Lombardia (14.4% *vs.* 5.4%).

The situation in Sicily, where private facilities prevail, is similar to that of Lazio; the situation in Piemonte, where there are no private facilities at all, is comparable with that of Lombardia. The percentage of patients treated at home or in limited care facilities is even higher, particularly if our programme at the S. Carlo Hospital is considered (Figure 8.3).

Limited care facilities, all run by public hospital dialysis units, differ in the degree of 'limitation of assistance' in the different areas of the country. Some of them, like that organized by my staff, work as 'minimal care' facilities. They are situated outside the hospital, usually in private buildings, and the patients, trained to be completely self-sufficient, take

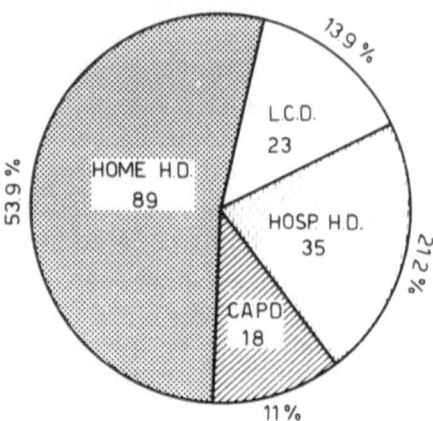

Figure 8.3 Distribution among different modalities of dialysis treatment of the total population of 165 patients on RDT at the S. Carlo Hospital at 15 February 1982
(HOME H.D = Home Haemodialysis; L.C.D. = Limited Care Dialysis; CAPD = Continuous Ambulatory Peritoneal Dialysis; HOSP. H.D. = Hospital Haemodialysis)

care of their own treatment, with the help of one nurse (a 'common partner' for all patients dialysing at the same time): no physician attends the treatment, and the medical supervision is usually carried out at fixed intervals during the month. Other satellite units are situated very far from the main unit, often in different towns. The choice of patients depends more on geographical location than on their attitude to self-care. The units have more staff, including also physicians attending the treatment and, in some cases, it is debatable whether they should be considered 'limited care' facilities at all.

Many people think that the quality of treatment given to patients in some regions, at least in profit-making institutions, is poorer in terms of survival and of clinical and social rehabilitation. ANED is continuously pointing this out and asking for closer control by the regional administrators. It is still a matter of controversy whether this low standard of treatment in private facilities is due more to the criteria of selection of patients or to the low level of assistance, necessary to make a profit, or to the organization of these facilities as free-standing out-patient centres, outside the hospital structure and, in practice, closed at night.

8.2.2 Selection policies

The criteria of selection vary quite a lot over the country in the different units, both public and private, and even from time to time within a single unit, according to the philosophy of the medical staff and to the changing availability of facilities in the surrounding territory. There is a general trend, however, to treat more aged patients and more patients with other

Table 8.3 Number of transplant units and patients in Italy at the end of 1980

	No. of transplant units	No. of patients transplanted	No. of dialysis patients transplanted in Italian units 1969–1980	1975–1980	transplanted abroad 1969–1980	1975–1980
Italy	11	1263	1263	863	891	729
Lombardia	3	569	492	317	77	46
Piemonte	0	0	52	40	89	76
Lazio	4	265	107	93	55	50
Sicilia	0	0	27	25	40	39

severe diseases, such as malignancies, diabetes, cardiovascular diseases, systemic collagen diseases, etc.

According to the data of ANED, the average age of the whole population of dialysed patients is increasing rapidly. In 1976, only 14.7% of patients were of retirement age (> 60 years for men, and > 55 years for women). Preliminary data for 1981 suggest that the percentage of these older patients is now over 30%. In Piemonte, one region of northern Italy, 57.2% of all patients on RDT at the end of 1981 were more than 50 years old. No doubt, this increase in the percentage of older patients in Italy is favoured by the more widespread use of CAPD. In a multicentre study, 67.8% of 197 CAPD patients, treated up to June 1981 by 14 units in northern Italy, were more than 50 years old.

8.3 RENAL TRANSPLANTATION

Let us now consider briefly the problem of transplantation in our country. There is no doubt that the proliferation of dialysis facilities and the large increase in the number of patients on RDT are also due to the inadequacy of transplant activity (Table 8.3). The inadequate development of a transplantation policy in Italy is due to many factors, such as:

(1) Legal obstacles (criteria for the definition and the establishment of cerebral death; consent of donor's next of kin; authorization necessary to remove a donor's kidneys).

(2) Indifference of the health care administrators in many regions.

(3) Resistance of physicians of different specialities, in particular of surgeons, to the 'transplant team' concept.

(4) Lack of co-operation by the medical staff of intensive care units in the provision of potential donors.

Between 1969 and the end of 1980 only 1263 patients were transplanted in Italy, 863 of them in the last 6 years, mainly using cadaver donors. In the same period, a further 729 dialysis patients were transplanted abroad, mainly in Belgium and in France. At the end of 1980 only 1107 were living in Italy with a functioning transplant. Again, the gap between northern Italy and the rest of the country is evident; out of 1263 patients transplanted in Italy, 925 were transplanted in hospitals in northern Italy, and nearly half (569) of these in Milan. No favourable trend towards an increase in the number and efficiency of transplant programmes is emerging from the data for 1981. The number of patients transplanted in Italy rose only from 240 in 1980 to 269 last year. However, a transplant unit has now started to operate in Piemonte after a long period of careful preparation and training. A bill that could remove some of the present legal obstacles, is being discussed by the Italian parliament and some regional administrations are studying measures to overcome the reluctance of the staff of intensive care units.

8.4 THE FUTURE

Some preliminary data from the ANED survey of the 1981 RDT programme in Italy are encouraging. They show that the percentage of home dialysis patients is slowly increasing and that the mushroom growth of facilities has ended. Some rational plans for the allocation of new facilities and the supervision of current programmes have been worked out by many regional health administrators, including those in Lazio and other regions of central and southern Italy. The increase in home dialysis is mainly due to the rapid growth of CAPD. In 1981 the number of patients treated with CAPD in Italy rose to 780, more than double the number being treated at the end of 1980 and about 5% of the total population of dialysis patients. Unfortunately, CAPD programmes are carried out exclusively by the dialysis units operating in public institutions and already involved in home haemodialysis. They are totally inadequate in central and southern Italy, where the private dialysis facilities are mainly located. At the end of 1981, 140 patients (30.4 per million of population) were being treated with CAPD in Piemonte, 229 (25.7 per million of population) in Lombardia and only 10 (2.0 per million of population) in Lazio. The future plan for this new mode of treatment was discussed at the last national congress of the Italian Society of Nephrology. The majority agreed that CAPD is cheaper than home haemodialysis and that it is easier to teach patients to perform at home. It was forecast that in a very short time more than 10–15% of dialysis patients would be treated in Italy with some type of continuous peritoneal dialysis. However, many of us emphasized the risk that a high percentage of patients will be forced to transfer from peritoneal dialysis to haemodialysis, due to unavoidable problems which limit the duration of CAPD, such as infections and metabolic complications and reduced permeability of the peritoneal membrane. This aspect must be accurately evaluated, to avoid the collapse of existing haemodialysis facilities and the consequent death of some patients. For these reasons, some nephrologists (and I am one of them) wonder whether it is correct to treat patients who are either very old or have severe complicating diseases and who were previously considered ineligible for dialysis.

8.5 ACKNOWLEDGEMENT

We are very grateful to dr. Franca Pellini Gabardini, Secretary of the "Associazione Nazionale Emodializzati" for consent to use the data of the ANED registry and for useful advice.

References

Associazione Nazionale Emodializzati (1981). Censimento dei servizi di dialisi e trapianto italiani al 31 dicembre 1980 (Milano, Arti Grafiche ERSER)

Blagg, C. R. and Scribner, B. H. (1980). Long-term dialysis: current problems and future prospects. *Am. J. Med.*, **68**, 633

Jacobs, C., Broyer, M., Brunner, F. P., Brynger, H., Donckerwolcke, R. S., Kramer, P., Selwood, N. H., Wing, A. J. and Blake, P. H. (1981). Combined report on regular dialysis and transplantation in Europe, XI, 1980. *Proc. Eur. Dial. Transplant Assoc.*, **18**, 2

9

Politics, morality and economics – are there choices?
L. Carter-Jones M. P.

9.1   INTRODUCTION

The decision that doctors face as to which patient should be treated by dialysis and which should receive a transplant, is basically not a medical one but a moral one. The doctor's exercise of clinical judgement is constrained by the lack of money for kidney units. This is the result of a choice regarding spending priorities within the National Health Service (NHS) and between the NHS and other areas of government spending. In turn, this choice is a political decision since politics is about choosing priorities and priorities are determined by political philosophy or, more simply, morality. Because we live in an imperfect world, we must also consider cost effectiveness.

Let me say at the outset that this painful debate on competing priorities in the NHS – on who lives and dies – should not be necessary and is caused by our present distorted sense of priorities. We are spending billions on weapons of mass destruction yet cutting back on services to save lives. However, I am a realist and, taking the economic and political situation as it is, I am going to argue that on both moral and economic grounds the treatment of kidney patients should be a priority. The prognosis, particularly for transplant patients, is much better than that for patients with other diseases whose treatment is much more expensive. So, kidney treatment gives value for money.

9.2   THE PRESENT SITUATION

I want first to review briefly the present situation. Britain is sixteenth in the European league for treatment of kidney failure. Spain and Cyprus treat more patients per head of population than we do. In 1979, 4500 patients were receiving treatment in the United Kingdom (UK) compared with 8000 in France, 6500 in Italy – countries with similar populations. During the period 1976–78, no new patients aged over 74 were accepted for treatment in the UK. In France the number was 115 and in West Germany 69. In the same years the UK accepted 29 new patients aged between 69 and 74 compared with 816 in France and 837 in West Germany. In the age range 45–65 years 1100 new patients were accepted in the UK compared with 1523 in France and 2136 in West Germany (*Hansard*, 1981d).

Each year in the UK there are about 2200 new cases of chronic renal failure yet in 1980 only 1373 new patients received treatment. That is, nearly one half died because there were no facilities to save them (*Hansard*, 1981c). Professor Cyril Chantler of Guy's Hospital, London, has stated that only 61 children under 15 received treatment in 1980 yet an estimated 90 suffered renal failure (quoted by Veitch, 1982).

9.3   THE BASIC PROBLEMS

The basic problems are a lack of money and a lack of kidneys available for transplantation.

9.3.1   Funds and value for money

Previous speakers (especially Dr Gabriel) have discussed the problems of funding. The report by the Medical Services Study Group of the Royal

College of Physicians (1981) on deaths from chronic renal failure in the West Midlands and Mersey Regions stating that no deaths occurred because of a shortage of machines was widely criticized. Published at the same time, a leading article in the *British Medical Journal* (1981) pointed out that several studies had shown clear relationships between the number of dialysis centres and the acceptance rate of patients into renal replacement programmes and the total number of patients having treatment. This situation was admitted to be very unsatisfactory by the Prime Minister in January 1981, and reiterated by the Minister of Health in reply to numerous parliamentary questions during 1981. The Prime Minister has said that it is 'not a satisfactory position, but there is a limit to the rate at which the NHS can increase provision, given the many calls on its resources' (*Hansard*, 1981a). But, particularly for a government determined to cut public expenditure, it would make economic sense to make more resources available for kidney treatment because, as I have said, in terms of prognosis related to cost, it is real value for money.

Many kidney diseases start in childhood. The development of ultrasound techniques means that congenital problems, such as obstruction in the urinary system, which cause progressive kidney damage, can be identified at about 32 weeks of pregnancy and arrangements can be made to start treatment at birth. The most common kidney problem in children is urinary tract infection, affecting 16 000 of 800 000 children born each year. Kidney failure occurs later in life in about 500 of these children. The damage is done by the age of five, so British researchers are now looking at ways of screening children. A simple urine test on one-year-olds could be the answer but the research is being inhibited by lack of money (Veitch, 1982). Recently, the Minister of Health said that the decision on screening was delegated to individual health authorities and that there was no definite evidence that routine screening was cost effective but research was continuing (*Hansard*, 1982c). We, therefore, have the opportunity to prevent death and the disability of a life harnessed to a machine – that is the human cost.

The latest DHSS figures for the financial cost (excluding drugs and investigations) are: £10 600 for a year's hospital haemodialysis; £7000 for home haemodialysis; £6200 for continuous ambulatory peritoneal dialysis (CAPD) and £5000 for a transplant (plus one year's follow-up) (*Hansard*, 1982c). These figures are somewhat lower than those given by Dr Pincherle (see Chapter 3).

Now let us compare the state of kidney treatment with that of heart transplants. The government gave £100 000 in 1980 to the Papworth unit at Everard, Cambridgeshire (although this was to top up a £300 000 grant from the Robinson Charitable Trust) – resources that had to be deducted from other areas of the NHS expenditure. The cost of a heart transplant is £17 000 but the prognosis for the patient is much worse than that for kidney patients. This is due to the availability of dialysis to sustain life if the transplanted kidney fails (Smith, 1979). Furthermore a patient who has been transplanted, or even treated by dialysis alone, has a longer survival than women who develop breast cancer and who, incidentally, have a much better prognosis than those (male or female) who develop cancer of the lung.

Quality of life is more difficult to assess than survival. Despite the necessity of drug treatment following a successful transplant the quality of life is infinitely superior to that achieved by dialysis in renal failure or the persistence of symptoms in those with heart failure. However, it may be that for those patients with renal failure who require to be treated by dialysis CAPD will give greater freedom than can be achieved by those tied to a haemodialysis machine.

9.3.2 Lack of available kidneys

Transplantation is the most effective and cheapest form of kidney treatment but there is a lack of available kidneys so that on 30 June 1981, 2079 patients were awaiting transplants in the UK (*Hansard*, 1981b). A significant factor in this situation was the effect of the BBC TV 'Panorama' programme on brain death on 13 October 1980. In the four weeks immediately following the programme the numbers of transplants dropped by half. In the period October 1979 to October 1980 a total of 784 transplants were performed in England compared with 596 in the twelve months October 1980 to September 1981, representing a decrease of about 24%.

However, it has been argued, for example, by Professor Bryan Jennett (quoted by Grist, 1981) that the fall-off in the number of transplants was due not to reluctance on the part of the public but the effect of the TV programme on doctors' attitudes. Professor Jennett believes that the supply of kidneys is affected mainly by the beliefs of the neurosurgeons and transplant surgeons in different units and by the fact that the application of the criteria for the diagnosis of brain death means a lot of extra work. Support for this view is indicated by the fact that some units did twice as many transplants after the programme as before, whilst others had reduced their activity by half.

The Medical Services Study Group of the Royal College of Physicians (1981) also found that doctors were reluctant to ask relatives' permission to remove kidneys, found the donation procedure time consuming and, because transplant surgery is recognized as a specialist field, were reluctant to remove kidneys, relying instead on one transplant team covering a wide area. The Minister of Health endorsed this view when he stated, in a recent parliamentary reply, that, 'evidence is that the supply of donor organs is limited mainly by the reluctance of many doctors to start the procedures necessary for transplantation. These procedures are set out in the code of practice on the removal of cadaveric organs for transplantation published in

1979 . . . the Department's Chief Medical Officer endorsed the recommendations on the implementation of the code made recently by the conference of Medical Royal Colleges . . . discussions are continuing with the profession to ensure that all doctors are made aware of the provisions of the code, the need for donor organs and the benefits that transplants bring to patients' (*Hansard*, 1982b). Certainly the BBC TV programme and the reply from the medical profession showed the real and even passionate division of professional opinion.

9.3.2.1 Ethical issues

The government is trying to increase kidney donations by promoting the donor card scheme and by the introduction, last year, of a new multi-donor card. But if we are to really tackle the problem of the lack of kidneys and the inadequate number of transplants, we must first tackle the need for a full public debate about the ethical issues involved. I would just like briefly to mention some of these issues and hope that the points will be taken up in later discussion.

9.3.2.2 The opting out scheme

At present the transplantation of human organs is regulated under the Human Tissues Act, 1961, whereby the hospital officer designated to authorize the removal of organs may do so if the deceased had previously recorded a wish to donate organs, by, for example, signing a kidney donor card. Or, if after he had made such reasonable enquiries as practicable, he had no reason to believe that the deceased would have objected or that any surviving relatives object to such removal (*Hansard*, 1980). I was a co-sponsor of the Bill introduced into parliament by Tam Dalyell on 23 October 1979. This would have allowed hospitals to take organs once clinical death was established unless the individual had contracted out during his/her lifetime, a fact which would be registered on a central computer. The Bill was introduced as a response to the lack of success of the kidney donor card in the early 1970s and the fact that kidneys are of no use one hour after death and an immediate decision is needed. The Bill was also in line with the French Caillavet law of 1976. The Bill failed to get a second reading in parliament but the issues have been raised subsequently several times.

9.3.2.3 Transplants from living donors

In the United States about half the transplants come from living donors, sometimes for money which is, of course, deplorable, but usually from a relative and the best results come from the use of well-matched organs taken from immediate relatives, the younger the better. But this can cause problems due to family pressure on potential donors and the ethical issues involved with a child or mentally handicapped person who cannot give valid consent. In the United States, courts have given permission for the removal of kidneys from dozens of children and mentally handicapped people (Smith, 1981). However, the new *BMA Ethical Handbook* (1979) came out strongly against kidney or other non-regenerative transplants from children. Most English lawyers believe that children cannot give valid consent to operations for someone else's benefit, nor can parents consent on their behalf.

However, this is an area of uncertainty. The law in Britain is confused regarding the removal of organs from patients dying in hospital and in obtaining permission from relatives. As I mentioned, the French have passed a law allowing immediate removal of organs for therapeutic or scientific purposes provided the person has not specifically objected during his/her lifetime. The Council of Europe have produced model laws which permit the donation of living organs but not for profit and also allow removal of non-regenerative organs from children and the mentally handi-capped. However, this applies only in families and the donor must have a capacity to understand what is intended and give consent.

I personally am very wary of transplants from children, but can appreciate the dilemma of parents with one healthy child and one needing a transplant. The legal situation in Britain needs to be resolved otherwise there is a danger of the growth of commercial trade in living organs as waiting lists get longer.

In the short term we could be doing much more to improve the situation. Firstly, there should be a really active campaign by the DHSS to promote donor cards. It is estimated that 15% of the population have indicated that they want to carry cards but only 10% have taken cards and only 1% actually carry them (Slapak, 1982). Secondly, there should be a computer bank system for potential donors. Recently the Minister of Health said he was not convinced this would significantly improve the situation and would cost £5 000 000 (*Hansard*, 1982a). However, I believe there are currently de-velopments towards establishing a computer bank and that a more realistic cost of this is £1 000 000 (on the basis of £50 000 for 2 600 000 people, Slapak, 1982). Not only does this make economic sense, but it will over-come the moral problem of having to ask relatives about donation at a time of grief and stress. I understand the computer bank would operate on a con-tracting in basis which I now prefer as being more ethically acceptable and practicable. I would suggest that, initially, in order to publicize and popularize the computer, prominent public figures, sports stars and pop idols should be persuaded to contract into the scheme.

9.4 SELECTION OF PATIENTS FOR TREATMENT

Finally, I want to touch on another matter which is a political, economic and moral problem and which concerns the great discrepancies between the number of patients receiving treatment in different regions. These figures reflect a number of factors including how long the service has been in existence and an amount of cross boundary referral but they also show – most importantly and disturbingly – varying criteria in the selection of patients. The variation in the 'mix' of criteria for medical rejection is clearly shown in the reports by the Medical Services Study Group (1981) and by Parsons and Lock (1980). But what really appalled and distressed me were the manifestly non-medical, social factors on which many decisions were made. It is true that in many cases social factors were combined with medical contraindications to treatment, such as 'widespread tuberculosis, spoke no English'. But I was shocked to see that patients were rejected because they were 'very unintelligent, dialysis/transplant not mentioned' – a 43-year-old person who lived 3 months after the onset of renal failure; 'mentally subnormal, only relative very elderly mother' – a 42-year-old who lived 1 year; another, 40 years old, had 'severe chronic psychiatric depression and personality disorder'. Finally, worst of all was a 4-year-old, denied treatment on the grounds of 'age and parent irresponsibility'.

Surely to select on mental subnormality and psychiatric grounds by themselves is to make an unwarranted value judgement on the worth of these people's lives. If an elderly or 'irresponsible' parent cannot cope with the patient's treatment this is a matter for social welfare, with the patient being taken into care – not for condemning a 4-year-old child to death.

The discrepancies between units in the selection of patients and the use of arguably, inadmissible social criteria, point to the need for a non-medical input into the decision and a right of appeal. The variations in the level of facilities between different Health Authorities indicate that the decision on priority and allocation of resources cannot be left entirely to the Area Authorities. National minimum guidelines should be laid down. But, the crux of the problem is that doctors are being forced to play God because of lack of courage by politicians.

Parliament and government must face up to and tackle the physical and moral issues involved in kidney transplant, firstly by clarifying the law on transplantation and, if necessary, passing new legislation and secondly, voting and earmarking extra funds.

I note that the Secretary of State has taken powers to intervene if Health Authorities are ignoring the Government's stated priorities for services to the elderly, mentally ill, mentally handicapped, children and maternity services. I do not want to divert resources from these areas, but we must make kidney treatment a priority with more funding in the form of specific grants. We should no longer tolerate the situation where whether or not a kidney patient lives or dies is a 'geographical gamble'. Morality and economy are on our side. We must make sure that the right choice is made.

References

B.M.A. Ethical Handbook (1979). British Medical Association, London
Hansard (1980). **4**, March, Col. 102
Hansard (1981a). **12**, Jan. Col. 469
Hansard (1981b). **17**, July, Col. 499
Hansard (1981c). **10**, Oct. Col. 449
Hansard (1981d). **16**, Oct. Col. 266
Hansard (1982a). **18**, Jan, Col. 54
Hansard (1982b). **23**, Feb. Col. 345
Hansard (1982c). **16**, March, Col. 98
Grist, L. (1981). Are some doctors pulling the plug? *General Practitioner.* 16, October, p. 73
Leading article (1981). Anonymous. Audit in renal failure: the wrong target. *Br. Med. J.*, **283**, 261
Medical Services Study Group of the Royal College of Physicians (1981). Deaths from chronic renal failure under the age of 50. *Br. Med. J.*, **283**, 283
Parsons, V. and Lock, P. (1980). Triage and the patient with renal failure. *J. Med. Ethics*, **6**, 173
Slapak, M. (1982). Personal communication.
Smith, T. (1979). *Times*, 28 Nov., p. 19
Smith, T. (1981). *Times Health Supplement*, 20 Nov., p. 19
Veitch, A. (1982). *Guardian*, 15 Jan., p. 4

Discussion

R. Stone (All Party Disablement Group): Is the reason known why the black population has a much higher incidence of renal failure?

K. D. Nolph: The incidence of hypertensive renal disease in particular is much higher in the black population. There may also be a higher incidence of other renal diseases but hypertension is one of the most striking.

Stone: Do we know the reason for that?

Nolph: No. We do not even know for certain the aetiology of most forms of hypertension. Differences in salt intake and in hereditary factors have been investigated. There have been a number of epidemiologic studies undertaken in the US trying to pinpoint the reason but there is no clear answer.

W. Cattell (St Bartholomew's Hospital): Prof Nolph gave us a preliminary report of the 12 centres' work from January to September. Could he tells us if these were new patients entering into the programme during that period?

Nolph: They were all patients in those programmes. We started follow-up monitoring in these centres on January 1 1981. The centres registered all their patients who were on CAPD at that time and during the year they entered all new patients. All patients were monitored. So we have some very experienced patients, in the group, plus all the new patients.

The life table analyses that we shall be doing will only include new patients who have been monitored from the moment they began CAPD. Our preliminary projections of life table analyses have numbers that are far too small for the registry as a whole and that is one of the reasons we have got to monitor all patients and follow them through a long enough period of time until the numbers on the registry reach significance. We are not quite there yet.

Cattell: The peritonitis rates in the two different analyses are totally different. In the 12-centre study there were already patients under treatment who may well have been self-selected in terms of infection rates.

Nolph: The figure of 1.9 episodes per patient-year was based on the pilot group of centres. The very first projection of a life table analysis was actually based on new patients only. The numbers are very small and I hesitate to show it other than as an example of what we intend doing. We shall be analysing all the complications in terms of both incidence and frequency distributions, and by life table analysis. We hope to do each one all three ways.

C. Wight (Addenbrooke's Hospital): I was speaking recently to a colleague of Professor d'Amico's working in Rome and discussing the difficulties of obtaining organs for transplantation. He gave me to understand that in some Italian intensive care units, should a potential or suitable donor die, there is a legal obligation to inform a member of the local transplantation team. Is that correct?

G. d'Amico: Our regulations permit us to take the kidneys of a potential donor if there is no refusal by the next of kin; but we have to ask their permission. The new laws would allow us to remove the kidneys if the patient himself had not refused before death, or if the next of kin did not formally object. But if there was written refusal that kidney could not be used.

Wight: I had understood that the physicians in the intensive care unit had a legal obligation to inform the renal unit of any potential donor.

d'Amico: Not at the moment, but the new national law should make this mandatory. Some regions already require this to be done, Lombardy for instance. But just the same they do not do it.

Wight: So I believe. But it is a way perhaps of obtaining more organs for transplantation.

d'Amico: It is certainly a way. Another way is to do away with the current regulation requiring every hospital to have a permit before any donor kidney can be taken. These permits are issued by the Ministry of Health and cause us considerable difficulty. We hope to do away with rules of this kind in the future.

K. Cole (Walsgrave Hospital): With an estimated 15000-plus patients on CAPD the incidence of episodes of peritonitis, catheter replacements and infection is proportionately low. Does the specialist CAPD nurse contribute to this factor? If the clinics are in general departments, similar to those which Dr Gabriel envisages in District General Hospitals, is training in CAPD techniques sufficient considering the longterm commitment that many dialysis nurses seem to display?

Nolph: The results that I showed reflect the results of a registry that is monitoring the activity in many different types of centre. Many of these centres are relatively inexperienced in peritoneal dialysis and are just starting. The registry also includes results from centres that have a long experience in intermittent peritoneal dialysis going on to CAPD. We can see that the results do differ in different centres and it is very difficult to know for sure which variables make the results better at one centre than another.

Mr Cole mentioned some aspects that I personally feel are very important. Patient selection is important. We have to recognize that each centre deals with different types of patients. Some centres have been very selective. Others have looked at CAPD as a relatively safe and easy therapy to start and have decided to approach selection by giving almost everybody a try at it and see how they do. This explains many of the dropouts. Many patients have recurrent episodes of peritonitis, but fortunately most of them do not become severely ill or have their life threatened, although that may happen.

Based on what I have seen, and my own experience, the success of a CAPD programme depends also on the team concept, and one of the most important members of that team is a very highly motivated skilled CAPD nurse. This should be a person who is very very mature in terms of dealing with all kinds of patients, someone who knows a lot about patient education amongst various levels of learners and someone who is very skilled at the CAPD technique as well. I strongly urge all centres to appoint only fulltime CAPD nursing personnel to the CAPD programme. People who work outside the CAPD team do not do as well. And a highly motivated nephrologist needs to be involved. Only a nephrologist understands the total medical care of a patient in any form of end-stage renal disease.

Dr Gabriel's proposal would be possible so long as highly skilled CAPD nurses were involved at the centre, and as long as the nephrologist was intimately involved.

I meet with our CAPD team twice a week and we review all the patients on a weekly basis, half of them on Tuesday mornings and the other half on Thursdays. We also include the dieticians and the social workers and that does contribute to the success.

We have found that general ward nurses should not participate at all in outpatient or inpatient care. When the patients come into the hospital we want only the team working with them or an IPD team that is highly skilled and highly trained. We really feel that only experienced PD personnel should be involved in the care of these patients.

d'Amico: I want to stress the necessity of having a trained team when starting CAPD. This is the most important factor in the results. But I am against Dr Gabriel's proposal, which is probably motivated by financial reasons, to give this task to the District Hospitals. The team for training patients to perform CAPD is very difficult to organize, but once organized it can work with quite a number of patients, training them, sending them home and taking care of them. There is no reason to have such teams well distributed geographically. The teams are also intended for emergencies and patients can travel, should it be necessary, to the hospital, which need not be too near their home.

For these reasons, if we want to avoid the results of hospitalization and the high dropout rate from CAPD noted in the EDTA survey, we shall have to distribute a number of training teams in various countries and put them to work.

F. M. Parsons (Leeds General Infirmary): We have heard that America is accepting approximately 80 new patients per million of population per annum with end-stage renal failure. Prof d'Amico quoted a figure of 55.7 in Italy. The UK is accepting only 24.6. There is a great discrepancy here. Mr Carter-Jones is obviously on our side. As he spoke there was no waving of order papers, the audience was quiet and there was no noise from the opposition. We do need help. Can he tell us how to get help?

Physicians have spoken up, they have also written in the weekly medical press and so on. Our voices seem to be falling on deaf ears, yet Mr Carter-Jones was so positive that we required help. How can he help us?

Carter-Jones: I do my best. I bet my bottom dollar that Ms Stone has been noting a few parliamentary questions that need to be asked already. It struck me that there was a very severe discrepancy and I should like to know why.

I am not always happy with the statistics that come out of the Department. It seems that they are reluctant to provide statistics. I was once told that I was causing them a lot of difficulty because I was asking so many questions and diverting resources away from the work that they were doing. I said to the Secretary of State, in all humility, in the presence of his civil servants that I was very sorry about this, but I thought that I was only asking the Secretary of State to share with me information that he already had.

I therefore became very worried, particularly in the perinatal campaign, that decisions could be made by Secretaries of State without the basic information. I can think of one episode in particular. I wanted to know the incidence of low-weight pre-term babies and I was told it would be counter-productive to find it. That was what I was told. Then one of the professors from Liverpool told me that they followed my questions in the House very carefully and they could not understand that reply because they could have provided the answer. So there can sometimes be a block in obtaining information.

If people do see the answers to questions in the House, and there are obvious discrepancies like the one that Dr Parsons has raised, they should let me or the All Party Group know and I am quite sure that we should be delighted to take it up.

C. S. Ogg: One of the problems that I see is to make sure that money that is intended to be used for treating people with renal failure is actually used for that purpose. As I understand it money leaves government for the Regions and is then sent to the local Health Authorities. In some regions that money is tied to specific clinical activities but in others it is not. In our own Region it is not. Regions say they can make policies but that it is up to local Health Authorities to implement those policies; they have a choice and they may choose to spend the money in other ways.

How can this be stopped?

Carter-Jones: This is very much a local matter, a matter for the committee responsible. There is the chance to make representation, particularly to the lay members of the Authority. The problem has to be faced at regional level. The medical profession may try sometimes to build empires and so some of the money may go, but that is really a description of medical politics. If there is a case to prove then one should get hold of the lay members and persuade them.

The other difficulty is that the Department, understandably in many ways and I come down on their side in this, are reluctant to give specific grants for special purposes. But every so often there comes a need for specific grants. If there is this discrepancy in acceptance rates between the UK and the States, and a discrepancy between our best and our worst, it really means that some Regions are performing abysmally, because we use average figures. The discrepancy between different areas is extremely high.

I think that that is a case for a specific and special grant and the case should be made, hopefully, by the people in the areas concerned.

The other thing I would go for, and the Department should consider this very carefully, is that there should be minimum standards laid down. If there are minimum standards then I would hope that those standards would be laid down by the medical profession, and I have no doubt in my own mind that they will lay down high minimum standards.

That is what I would go for.

J. Michael (Queen Elizabeth): What is Mr Carter-Jones's understanding of the legal position of a patient denied treatment for reasons of lack of funding.

Carter-Jones: I do not really know and I think the case should be tested sometime by the Ombudsman. It would be wrong of me to even pretend I know that answer but it is the sort of thing that wants testing, and the sooner the better in my view.

With regard to the non-delivery of services, RADAR is presently making an effort to see that certain provisions of the Alf Morris Act are implemented on the grounds that there are legal rights within the Act. I have a funny feeling, it is only a hunch and a politician's hunch, that if it were challenged the patient could win, and win substantially on the ground that the service should be provided to him or her. But that is only a hunch and I should like to see it tested.

Stone (All Party Disablement Group): The Government is really set against making specific grants and laying down national minimum standards, although it is significant that they have made a statement about Health Authorities not carrying out the government's priorities. They do intend to lay down some minimum guidelines for maternity services.

But what happens to the money is basically a local decision and political activity at that level is important. Those who work in these fields must work through their Community Health Councils, they must get on to the local MPs in the vicinity of the Area Health Authority and get them to ask questions in Parliament about the level of renal services for that particular area and have that publicized in the local press. Thus they should put the Chairman of the District Authority on the mat and ask for some sort of explanation.

It is only through that sort of local pressure, applying local publicity, and getting MPs involved, that a difference is made. MPs in the All Party Group can beaver away at the Minister for longterm changes and extra funding, but for a more immediate result work has got to be done at the local level.

R. F. M. Wood (John Radcliffe Hospital): I think it is most impressive that we have people in Parliament who have such a clear grasp of the problems of dialysis and transplantation.

I should like to ask about the kidney donor card scheme. Public opinion does not really favour a contracting out scheme and there is more support for a contracting in scheme, as is shown by people carrying a kidney donor card. It is unfortunate that more people do not carry kidney donor cards and I suspect that part of the reason is that a card at present has no legal standing.

Is there any chance of a Bill in Parliament in the near future to give the kidney donor card legal standing which would enable us, as transplant surgeons, to proceed with cadaver nephrectomy without having to approach relatives and go through the whole distressing procedure even though the patient had a signed donor card.

Carter-Jones: We may need legislation because of the legal and ethical issues involved. Similar measures have been introduced primarily by Private Members' Bills, and though the Chronically Sick and Disabled Persons Act is quite complex and very often considered to be mandatory, it is permissive in many ways and it had to be done by backbenchers.

I would guess that this sort of legislation – I may be wrong and somebody may be bold enough to pick it up – is not suitable for private members' time, because if the government want to block it they would block it. Really we shall have to persuade government to introduce the bill.

All sorts of things were said about the contracting out bill introduced by Tam Dalyell.

I am quite sure that the All Party Group would support some contracting in scheme. It may be worth putting it to the Government to see if they would consider doing it.

G. Pincherle (Department of Health and Social Security): The donor card is a legal document. A surgeon is totally entitled in law to take out a kidney on the strength of a signed donor card unless there is any reason to believe that the patient might have changed his or her mind between signing it and the time of death. The fact that most surgeons also ask the next of kin is an ethical point with which I would be in complete agreement, but it is an ethical point not a legal one. Indeed, were we to have a contracting in system with a computer, which the patient might have notified 2 or 3 years previously, I am not so sure that that would be sufficient legal authority to take out the kidney because the patient might well have changed his mind in that time, whereas the fact that he was carrying the card on him would be *prima facie* evidence that he had not changed his mind.

We have had questions on the right to treatment. Under the NHS Act as I understand it there is no right to treatment. This was tested a year or two ago in the courts when someone sued the Secretary of State because there was a four-year waiting list for hip replacement operations and lost.

G. Oreopoulos: In Ontario we have had donor cards for many years and these have been very successful. Almost every citizen of Ontario has one. But, we have found that we can only use it rarely and it has not been very successful in increasing the supply of kidneys. We have found it of greater use as a public relations exercise and a means of increasing awareness. Continued pressure, through, for example, the media, to make the public aware that, at a critical moment, someone may ask them for a kidney is more important than the card. We have found that whether relatives have heard about or have discussed kidney transplantation previously is of more importance than whether the victim had a donor card.

Nolph: When we renew our driver's licences we all have the option to sign a donor card. It is on the back of the driver's licence.

We also find that surgeons and doctors still want to ask the family, and very rarely would they transplant against the wishes of the family. So it has had the same impact, although everybody has it on the back of their driver's licence.

Carter-Jones: I am worried that people at the end of the day are not carrying their donor cards. I would agree that the DHSS has not made enough effort because really people ought to carry them.

But there is something rather positive in going out of one's way to get one's name on to a computer. The only reason to object seems to be that someone might change his mind. That seems to be a very simple administrative problem. People who want to get taken off the computer can get taken off the computer – and they can declare it. Someone who changes his mind will have thought long about it and said that it was not for them. If they go to that extent I am quite sure they would take the trouble to get themselves removed.

The case of the hip replacement and the four-year wait has been mentioned. It is not very pleasant for the patient waiting for a hip replacement. There would be rather more emotion raised, and I am not averse to emotion now and then, if the cause is right. It would not be a bad thing to sue the Secretary of State because by the time the case got to court the patient would be dead and the point would have been proved.

Ogg: We are now members of the EEC and I believe there is a provision whereby if a form of treatment is not available in one member country but is in another, the patient can be sent to the country where that form of treatment is available, for instance from England and Italy. And then the Italians might be invited to bill the Health Authority from which the patient came.

Am I right in this?

Carter-Jones: I do not know the answer, but it is a good idea.

Pincherle: Strictly speaking Dr Ogg is right, but I suspect that not many patients would be willing to move lock, stock and barrel to Italy, although some might.

We have had a case of someone having a transplant carried out in Belgium under these arrangements.

It is a little bit like buying a new car!

S. N. Taber (EDTNA): Should we not be putting the *Panorama* programme into transplant history? I though we had decided about 6 months ago that our brain death criteria were perfectly all right, they had been amended. The donor card scheme is an excellent idea. The computer opting in scheme is an excellent idea. But, are we not back to the apathy of medical and nursing staff?

I do not know whether Mr Carter-Jones has heard of the role of the transplant co-ordinator. What does he feel about such personnel? We are not an organization; there are about five in post at the moment. Their purpose is professional education, with 25% their time spent on educating the general public.

Cattell (St Bartholomew's Hospital): To come back to funding, we are all agreed that the UK replacement programme is under-funded and that there must be additional sums of money and possibly more efficient uses of available money. I was very attracted by Prof Oreopoulos's closing slides in which he examined the question of how we spent our money, whether we spent it on useless investigations, or whether as a group we demonstrated that we were efficient and used our money to good purpose.

However, there is a snag in the United Kingdom. The most recent reorganization has created yet another problem in that renal replacement is primarily a Regional service, by which I mean that within the United Kingdom we are now broken down into some six hundred plus districts whereas the replacement service, the unit, provides for perhaps 15 or 16 of these Districts.

If money is allocated, additional money, or if there are pressures for more cost-effective use to be made of one's own money, this is seen within the budget of a District, not a Region. Furthermore, that District has its pressures in terms of mentally handicapped, maternal care, etc. And if I run my own dialysis programme efficiently and I save money, I have no access to that money and it will be spent on someone else. Therefore there is a disincentive to be cost-effective in renal replacement because the money will be pinched.

During the time of the previous government there was an allocation of funds for extra kidneys, the famous kidney machines. It was eventually decided that this money should be handed out to various Regional Health Authorities. One Regional Health Authority in London received their allo-cation of funds for additional facilities for dialysis, or renal replacement. How-ever, as the months went by they wondered what had happened to the money. It eventually transpired that it had actually been used on geriatrics and mentally handicapped. Both of these are extremely worthy areas, but it is this sort of problem that worries us.

We do not have the same control over our budgets in the UK as occurs in Toronto and in Columbia, and, although the DHSS may not like it, they will have to seriously examine a separate Regional budget for renal replace-ment. It is no good saying that this is something that will be handed down to the grass roots. What happens in these circumstances is that regional treasurers have power without responsibility. They decide on a figure and they say 'there you are boys'. There is no control as to whether any sum they allocate will ever benefit one patient with kidney failure.

I would suggest that integral to providing more money we must have a much better budgeting system for these services.

Carter-Jones: If money is specifically allocated and treasurers have got away with it then I am surprised. It really means that the audit section has fallen down rather badly in doing its work. One of the things the Civil Service is supposed to be very good at doing is seeing that money is spent on the purpose for which it was allocated. I wonder whether specific grants have been made.

There is, I understand, a special investigation being conducted on whether the various Area Health Authorities and other authorities are spending wisely and getting value for money. It may well be that in this analysis of expenditure in the Health Service, this could be one of the things they could take into account. But the question of 'misappropriation' of resources allocated for specific purposes does not normally come to

Parliament. It is a useful question to answer but I should have thought that it was really a matter for the DHSS auditors.

Pincherle: As Mr Carter-Jones said, the Department does not like earmarking money. Money was given to the Regional Health Authorities with a 'moral' earmark but not a legal earmark. Whilst the Health Authority may not have acted over-ethically in using the money for geriatrics or something else it was not acting illegally and there was no question of misappropriation.

Cattell: What a splendid piece of balderdash! If Dr Pincherle can stand up and try to justify what Mr Carter-Jones correctly describes as the misappropriation of funds in that manner, it is a deplorable situation. The money was allocated by the Secretary of State primarily because of a great deal of effort and lobbying to raise funds to help kidney patients. Both the Chancellor and the Secretary of State at that time specifically indicated that this was the purpose for which that money was to be spent.

I am not qualified to understand the finer points of the legality in the Department of Health, but Dr Pincherle's answer is wholly unacceptable.

D. Benoliel (National Federation of Kidney Patients' Associations): We are talking about the carrying of donor cards. We all appreciate very much Mr Carter-Jones's support for us, but I would wish to support Dr Oreopoulos's view and Ms Taber's view that the value of carrying a donor card is a public relations exercise. It is a very valuable one and the DHSS has probably gone as far as it can in doing that. The Department should now be turning its efforts to educating doctors. What Ms Taber said about the role of the transplant co-ordinator is very true.

Ogg: The time has come to draw the Session to a close. I have enjoyed it very much, particularly the stimulating discussion.

SESSION THREE

The State of the Art in the United Kingdom
Chairman:
A. C. Kennedy

Chairman's Introduction
A. C. Kennedy

This Session falls into two parts and in my remarks I shall deal with them separately.

In the first part of the Session we are to hear accounts of the current situation in the United Kingdom as regards transplantation, haemodialysis and CAPD. We shall hear what we are achieving, what the problems are and what might be done to improve the situation. Inevitably there will be some contrasts with what we have heard in respect of Canada, the United States, Italy and elsewhere.

The United Kingdom approach since the mid-sixties has been characterised by tight budgetary control from the Central Health Departments, exercised essentially by strict control in the number of units providing services and in the staffing of these units. It is my belief that these units are very fully extended, certainly in respect of dialysis, that they are very efficiently run by a hardworking and very loyal staff, and that they have been extremely aware of the paramount importance of pursuing policies enabling the greatest number of patients to be treated by the most economical methods. For example, as regards transplantation, the cheapest form of treatment, the number of transplants we do is relatively much higher than in the United States or in Italy, and indeed the number of patients with a functioning transplant in the United Kingdom now exceeds the number of patients on home dialysis. This is good, but we could do better. We could do more if only there was a more plentiful supply of kidneys.

As regards haemodialysis, the UK has been the pace setter in respect of the proportion of patients being dialysed at home. Again a very cost-effective approach born out of the absolute necessity for units to move patients out from the hospital as the limited number of units became full to overflowing. I doubt if we can really improve our performance here as we are probably at the limit of the percentage of patients we can usefully transfer to home.

As regards CAPD, we have seized with enthusiasm and with relief this new quite simple and relatively cheap form of treatment and we are exploiting it vigorously. It has provided us with a welcome expansion point in the past 2 or 3 years, but I suspect that we may soon be in danger of reaching a plateau in the number of patients on CAPD because of pressure on available back-up beds to handle those patients who develop complications.

How much further do we wish to go to increase our intake of new patients, which at present is around 25 patients per million of population, and how much further can we afford to go without prejudicing health care elsewhere? Being entirely realistic I do not think we should seek or could hope to have a situation where there is absolutely no selection process other than a diagnosis of chronic renal failure. Benefit cannot be solely judged in terms of prolongation of life. There is also quality of life. Selection is not simply a question of age although obviously major infirmities, physical or mental, or both, are more likely to be present in those of very advanced years. My own view is that we should concentrate our energies on obtaining sufficient additional resources to bring our annual new intake up to 35–40 patients per million of population in all regions of the country without further pressure on our existing units. This would be a very considerable advance on what we have at present, and it is after all the target figure that we nephrologists gave the Central Health Department many many years ago, and one which I believe they accepted in principle. It would require quite considerable additional expenditure unless we were extraordinarily successful in increasing the number of transplants carried out.

So much for my very brief, necessarily over-simplified opening remarks. I shall be interested to hear how our speakers approach this topic.

10

The current United Kingdom transplant situation
R. Y. Calne

10.1 INTRODUCTION

When I first became interested in transplantation in 1959 patients with renal failure had no chance of treatment. They were made as comfortable as possible and died. In 1960, two notable events occurred; an effective immunosuppressive drug, namely azathioprine was introduced and Scribner showed that an arteriovenous shunt could be made to last a long time and allow a patient to be rescued from uraemia by repeated dialysis. Although from time to time there has been rivalry between transplantation and dialysis, it is now clear that they are complementary and whilst dialysis is a relatively safe procedure it imposes serious restrictions on the patient. He must be careful how much he drinks, watch his salt intake, and may suffer from complications from the arterio-venous fistula requiring revision of the anastomosis. He will have a chronic anaemia and worst of all, he has to be both physically and psychologically wedded to a complicated machine for several hours, two or three times a week. Maintaining a patient on dialysis is expensive in equipment but more so in terms of the medical, nursing and technical staff who support the patient, even though these costs are reduced when dialysis is conducted at home.

10.2 IMMUNOSUPPRESSION

Successful renal transplantation has the great advantage for the patient of making him completely independent and fully rehabilitated to a degree that is not possible with maintenance dialysis. If a transplant comes from an identical twin indefinite function is to be expected unless the primary renal disease attacks the transplanted kidney. Results are nearly as good if the kidney is given by a brother or sister who is matched for the main human tissue groups and there is a one in four chance of two siblings having the same group. A patient with such a well matched kidney will still require immunosuppressive drug treatment but rejection is unusual. Recipients of kidneys from other close blood relatives do better than from unrelated dead donors where approximately 50% of grafts function at one year, although the patient survival is nearer 80% because of the availability of dialysis if the kidney fails.

10.2.1 Azathioprine and steroids

Recipients of kidney grafts must be treated with potentially toxic drugs in order to control the natural rejection of the body to the graft. Although many agents have been used in the past, the sheet-anchor of immuno-suppressive treatment is still the combination of azathioprine and steroids. Azathioprine has an inhibitory effect on the bone marrow and may cause a fall in the number of circulating white cells and platelets, increasing susceptibility to infection. However, the drug is usually well tolerated and not too difficult to control. Serious side-effects are now not common.

Corticosteroids (cortisone and prednisolone) have well known and unpleasant side-effects unless the dosage is very low. Most patients requiring sufficient steroids to prevent rejection develop side-effects, particularly the moon face of Cushing's syndrome and a general increase in weight. In children, corticosteroids inhibit growth and the moon-faced, stunted child may find it very difficult to lead a happy integrated life with other school children. Corticosteroids may also damage joints and can cause severe destruction of the hips. There are many other side-effects but these are the most unpleasant.

10.2.2   Cyclosporin A

Some four years ago cyclosporin A, a new immunosuppressive drug, became available for investigation. It is quite different from any other agent so far used and, like many antibiotics, is the product of a fungus. In fact it has weak antibiotic properties itself, but it has a very powerful effect on the inhibition of graft rejection. Unfortunately, the drug can cause temporary damage to the kidney, especially when it is used in large doses and it is therefore difficult to use. However, with experience the results of kidney grafting from unrelated dead donors using this drug have improved to around 80% functional survival of the transplant at a year; this figure should be compared to that of about 50% in patients treated with azathioprine and steroids.

It is likely that new derivatives of cyclosporin A will be developed in a similar way to the remarkable derivatives produced from the original penicillin, but even with the presently available drug it is clear that cyclosporin A has resulted in an important advance in treatment of patients with organ grafts. It has been used successfully in recipients of livers, pancreases, hearts and even hearts and lungs. The stage should be set now for a general increase in organ grafting with the expectation of improved longterm survival. One of the most attractive features of cyclosporin A is that patients do not usually require longterm corticosteroids as well and some of the most unpleasant side-effects of immunosuppressive treatment can therefore be avoided. Because of the steroid-sparing effect we have started transplanting children and a baby of 18 months transplanted with a kidney from an unrelated dead donor is now doing well 2 years later with normal renal function.

10.3   THE AVAILABILITY OF TRANSPLANTS

Patients with good functioning grafts can engage in all normal activities including competitive sports. The cost of a transplant is obviously much less than maintenance dialysis. In a Health Service which is short of resources the argument for transplanting as many patients as possible is very strong, but this also applies to countries such as the United States where more money is available for health care. If treatment of patients with renal failure by a combination of dialysis and transplantation is effective then the 2000 or so new cases who require treatment each year in the UK will for the most part survive, so that the size of the pool of patients under treatment increases to a considerable degree each year, demanding an increasing share of the limited resources devoted to the Health Service. The argument to increase the number of transplants is strong, but this can only be done if more donor kidneys become available.

It is ironic that at a time of improvement in a therapeutic endeavour, the number of donors which has always been grossly inadequate has in fact actually fallen in the UK. Not one of the thirty transplant centres are fully occupied and most work at around half their potential capacity, a dreadful waste. The reason for the shortfall in donors is complicated, but the main setback that occurred following the BBC TV programme 'Panorama' (13 October 1980) was tragically obvious. The enormous power of television undermined the confidence of the public in the integrity of the medical profession and raised doubts that organs were being removed from people who were not dead. A second BBC television programme was aimed at permitting a more fair debate on the subject, since the first programme was like a trial in a totalitarian country with a powerful case for the prosecution, no defence and witnesses that were irrelevant to the proceedings. Just before the end of the debate on the second programme, one of the opponents of the British criteria of brain death, said that he knew of two patients who fulfilled the criteria of brain death and yet recovered completely. This fanned the fires of doubt and mistrust. His complete withdrawal of this statement in a letter to the *Lancet* received virtually no publicity and so the harm was done. It is very sad because public opinion had moved increasingly to a charitable attitude towards those suffering from kidney disease and other conditions where an organ graft can save a young life. Many sections of the medical profession were prepared to help in organ donation, despite the fact that this requires considerable extra work on behalf of a patient they may not have seen and often involves prolonged consultation with colleagues and the relatives of the dead person, which may be distressing for both parties. Some doctors have preferred not to co-operate in organ donation and it is remarkable how the spirit of charity in this respect varies from one

Table 10.1 Variation in procurement and use of kidney transplants in adjacent Regions in the UK, 1978–1981

	Patients receiving kidneys	*Kidney donors*	*Number of donors per patient transplanted*
Norfolk	54	26	0.48
Hertfordshire Essex Lincolnshire Buckinghamshire	49	9	0.18
Suffolk	35	22	0.63
Cambridgeshire	24	68*	2.83
Bedfordshire	15	17	1.13

* Two from Peterborough

hospital to another and even between different consultants within the same hospital.

Kidney transplantation is performed in Regional Centres which have a responsibility to undertake transplants on patients coming from hospitals all over the Region. It would not seem unreasonable to expect co-operation in organ donation from all the hospitals in the Region, whose patients with renal failure are receiving kidney transplants from the transplant centre. But, as can be seen from Table 10.1, there is a marked variation and some hospitals benefit greatly from the number of their patients who are transplanted, but contribute very little to organ donation, despite the fact that doctors from the Regional Centre are prepared to go out at any time of the day or night to any part of the Region and remove kidneys.

10.3.1 The law

The law in the UK on removal of kidneys from dead people has never been tested. It was framed in 1961 before organ transplantation was performed. It is a mixture of an 'opting in' and an 'opting out' system, so that if the deceased's wishes are known and favourable towards organ donation as indicated, for instance, by the fact that he carried a donor card, then it is lawful to remove his organs without any further consultation. If the deceased's wishes are not known, then the next of kin must be approached, not to ask permission, but to determine what would have been the wishes of the deceased. Despite this, the interview usually turns out to be a request for permission. If the next-of-kin cannot be approached because, for example they do not exist, it is lawful for the organs to be removed provided there is no objection from the coroner. Most cases suitable for organ donation come under the coroner's jurisdiction, being accident victims or cases of sudden death from, for example, cerebral haemorrhage. The coroner can order an autopsy which involves removing all the organs from the body at least for inspection, without any objection from the relatives or anyone else. He must also satisfy himself that organ removal for transplantation will not interfere with his duty, which is to make sure that the cause of death does not involve any criminal act. Most coroners are now sympathetic towards the needs of transplantation.

Under the present Human Tissue Act it may be very difficult for the doctors who have cared for the deceased to discuss the question of organ donation with the relatives in time for the organs to be of any use, as they must be removed immediately after death. This is particularly the case in victims of road traffic accidents and especially so when they are children. Under such circumstances the relatives may not be able to even comprehend what the doctors say. Yet frequently they will telephone later or even write to say they wished the organs to be used to help someone else. A change of the law to a complete contracting out system might avoid causing this kind of distress. It would be assumed that consent for organ removal had been given unless the name of the deceased, or the family name in the case of a child, had been recorded in a central information computer. It seems unlikely that such a change in the law will come about in the UK in the near future, although legislation on these lines has been passed in a number of countries such as France, Denmark and Austria.

10.4   THE FUTURE

What then can be done to improve the present unhappy state of affairs? First and foremost the confidence of the public needs to be restored in the medical profession. The criteria of brain death accepted in the UK have been tested in many hundreds of cases and there has never been an error provided the fairly simple clinical conditions are met. The purpose of having these criteria is not primarily to provide organs for transplantation, but to avoid continuing to ventilate a corpse, which cannot help the dead person and which will cause only distress to the relatives and nursing staff in attendance. Since the adoption of these criteria the care of patients with brain damage throughout the country has improved and the medical profession is far more aware of how to care for these cases on ventilators. The BBC having caused so much damage to sick people has an obligation to try to put things right by suitable programmes demonstrating what is done in transplantation and what can be achieved. Hospitals which wish to have patients treated by transplantation should fulfil their obligation to help with organ donation so that more patients can be treated. There should be more than enough organs for transplantation purposes from victims of road traffic accidents, brain haemorrhages and primary tumours of the brain. The plight of those needing treatment is well known to the public and profession alike and surely this will restore a charitable attitude to organ donation.

11

Haemodialysis: the current situation in the United Kingdom
J. Walls

11.1 INTRODUCTION

At present regular haemodialysis is the commonest method of treatment for end-stage renal disease in the UK, but despite the full committment of individual renal units, the UK still lags behind many other European nations in achieving the acceptance rate for new patients of 45 per million population per annum, a figure suggested by several studies (Dombey *et al.*, 1975; Laing, 1980). The rapid growth in the number of patients treated by continuous ambulatory peritoneal dialysis (CAPD) may go some way to redressing this discrepancy, although there is anxiety regarding the 'drop out' rate from CAPD, which could further stress existing haemodialysis facilities (Wing, 1982). During the past five years a number of developments have occurred in haemodialysis therapy throughout the world. These can be divided into changes in patient management and of dialysis techniques. In addition, some major clinical problems have evolved and in some cases solutions have been offered.

11.2 MANAGEMENT

11.2.1 Provision of facilities

Since the mid-1960s, home haemodialysis has been the goal for most renal units in the UK, thereby allowing a single unit of 10–12 beds/stations to cope with up to 150 patients. This trend has continued in the UK throughout the 1970s and the development of large hospital-based out-patient dialysis facilities has not occurred for a variety of reasons including finance and the prevention of hepatitis, etc. In 1972, the USA which was developing home dialysis programmes in parallel with European countries, changed direction with a decrease in this mode of therapy in favour of minimal care or satellite dialysis units. Such units provide a variable degree of nursing, technical and medical care, relying on the patient's ability to self-dialyse. Recently there has been a slow development of minimal care dialysis units in the UK (Table 11.1) with most units centred around either Merseyside or London. Many of these units were financed from 'charitable sources', some having a low patient usage rate, and only a handful are planned for the future.

Table 11.1 'Minimal care' dialysis in UK, 1982

Region	No. units	No. beds	No. patients	Units planned
Mersey	4	16	32	4
London	3	16	17	1
N. W. England	2	8–10	12–14	0
W. Midlands	1	4	6	0
Wessex	1	4	3	0
'Rest'	0	0	4	Possible 7

11.2.2 Dialyser use

The past few years has seen a steady decline in the use of non-disposable parallel flow dialysers and coil dialysers in Europe with a reciprocal growth in the use of disposable parallel flow and hollow fibre dialysers. Similar trends have been seen in the UK although they have developed at a slower rate. In 1974, 68.1% of all dialyses in the UK used a Kiil type dialyser but in 1981 this had fallen to 31.5% with disposable parallel flow and hollow fibre dialysers contributing approximately 30% each. These figures, and comparable figures for Europe are shown in Table 11.2. However, unlike Europe, most UK renal units re-use disposable dialysers, in some cases up to six times.

The duration of dialysis has slowly decreased during the past 5 years to between 12 and 18 hours per week, usually on a thrice weekly basis. The patient's body weight appears to have little effect on dialysis time or whether dialysis is performed in hospital or at home.

Table 11.2 Dialyser use in UK and Europe, 1981

Dialyser	UK	Europe
Non-disposable 'plate'	31.5%	3.1%
Disposable 'plate'	30.7%	34.1%
Coil	8.8%	16.4%
Hollow fibre	29%	34.1%
Haemo filters	0	1.3%

11.2.3 Problems

11.2.3.1 Aluminium intoxication

Throughout the 1970s there was widespread recognition of two clinical syndromes associated with haemodialysis, dialysis encephalopathy and fracturing osteodystrophy. The incidence of these syndromes shows a wide regional variation, i.e. 38.9% of patients at a renal unit in Glasgow had dialysis encephalopathy and up to 75% of patients using softened water in Newcastle had fracturing osteodystrophy (Parkinson et al., 1979). Similar reports also emanated from North America (Alfrey et al., 1976; Posen et al., 1972). The possibility that a water-borne contaminant, namely aluminium, might be the aetiological agent was suggested by the studies of Flendrig et al. (1976) and of Platts et al. (1977). Further confirmation that high water concentrations of aluminium were to blame was demonstrated by the epidemiological study of Parkinson et al. (1979) which showed a strong positive correlation between the percentage incidence of dialysis encephalopathy and the mean water concentration of aluminium. A similar significant correlation with fracturing osteodystrophy was also demonstrated.

It would therefore appear that aluminium accumulates in patients on haemodialysis and more recent studies (Hodge et al., 1981) have demonstrated a positive transfer of aluminium from dialysis fluid into the patient occurring at concentrations above 15 to $18\,\mu g/l$ (mean $14\,\mu g/l$). As aluminium is not removed by water softeners (commonly used to remove calcium from tap water) better treatment of raw water for dialysis by reverse osmosis would appear essential in areas with high concentrations of aluminium in water (Ward et al., 1978), together with regular monitoring of both water and serum aluminium concentrations to prevent accumulation of aluminium. A dialysis fluid concentration of aluminium of less than $50\,\mu g/l$ is necessary, and possibly less than $20\,\mu g/l$, although the latter is difficult to achieve as commercial dialysate currently available in the UK may contribute up to $15\,\mu g/l$. The significance of serum aluminium levels requires further evaluation.

The effects of other trace metals or contaminants in water supplies is under continual review and other clinical syndromes may well become apparent with time.

11.2.3.2 *Malignancy*

Recognition of the increasing incidence of *de novo* malignancy in uraemic patients both on conservative and haemodialysis therapy, has occurred in the past 5–7 years (Matas et al., 1975; Miach et al., 1976; Sutherland et al., 1977 and Herr et al., 1979). Similar data from the EDTA Registry (Brynger et al., 1980) has shown a six-fold increase in the death rate due to malignancy in young adult dialysis patients compared to that of the general population. This trend also exists for middle aged and older patients but to a lesser extent. In addition, the presence of cysts and adenomas in end-stage kidneys of dialysis patients has been described (Dunnill et al., 1977) and some haemodialysis patients have died from disseminated malignancy originating from a renal primary (Walls, 1982). These observations have implications with regard to dialysing older patients and the effects of immunosuppression post-transplantation.

11.3 VASCULAR ACCESS

The arteriovenous shunt, which allowed regular haemodialysis to be established in the early 1960s has been mainly superseded by the arteriovenous fistula and certain types of prosthesis such as bovine carotid and PTFE grafts. A major development in vascular access occurred in 1979 with the introduction of a sub-clavian catheter which could be used in the single needle mode (Uldall et al., 1979). The position of such catheters allows full patient mobility even as an out-patient, and the technique is of inestimable benefit in the management of new patients presenting in end-stage renal failure, patients with chronic renal failure awaiting the maturation of an arteriovenous fistula, patients with acute renal failure, occasional patients on CAPD who require temporary haemodialysis because of severe peritonitis and patients receiving plasmapheresis. The catheter is simply placed under local anaesthesia using a check X-ray to ensure correct positioning. Inevitably, with a new technique, some complications occur including those due to incorrect positioning and perforation of the sub-clavian vein; however these are invariably due to faulty techniques or operator error. This method of access can be used for several weeks or months, if the catheter is replaced at regular intervals to prevent the occurrence of septicaemia. Clot formation within the catheter is prevented by regular daily flushing with heparinized saline. This development has allayed many of the fears of patients with troublesome vascular access and further modifications such as the use of a double lumen catheter to improve blood flow rates are imminent.

11.4 TECHNIQUES OF DIALYSIS

The trend to shorter dialysis schedules as advocated by Cambi et al. (1974), whilst desirable in some aspects such as shortening the dialysis time for the patient, and allowing more patients to be treated on the same equipment, has led to problems associated with rapid fluid removal. Rapid ultrafiltration during short dialysis produced symptomatic hypotension in 20 to 30% of haemodialysis patients increasing both their morbidity and mortality and the workload of the renal unit nursing staff. This topic has recently been reviewed by Shaldon (1981). A variety of new techniques has evolved in an attempt to circumvent this problem.

11.4.1 Haemofiltration

Haemofiltration as an alternative to conventional haemodialysis was introduced by Henderson et al. (1967) but has only gained popularity as a mode of therapy for uraemia in the past half decade. The usual method is to remove up to 20 litres of ultrafiltrate per treatment with post-dilutional fluid replacement with a modified Ringer-lactate solution (Quellhorst et al., 1978). Although large volumes of fluid are removed and replaced during haemofiltration the incidence of symptomatic hypotension is less than that in the same patients on standard acetate haemodialysis. It is also claimed that haemofiltration has a number of other advantages over standard haemodialysis in addition to better patient tolerance (Schneider et al., 1977) (Table 11.3). This procedure is practised mainly in Germany and France. In

Table 11.3   Haemofiltration

Advantages	Disadvantages
Improved large molecule clearance	Possible depletion syndromes
Shorter treatment times	Hospital based
Better patient tolerance	Cost – filters
Improved hypertension control	infusion fluid
Improvement in hyperlipidaemia	

1981 only the occasional patient in the UK was treated by haemofiltration and it is difficult to assess whether the claims of other workers justifies the increased cost of this type of treatment.

11.4.2   Bicarbonate dialysis

Since 1964, acetate has replaced bicarbonate as the buffering agent in dialysis fluid but in 1977 the Seattle group (Graefe *et al.*, 1977) demonstrated that the incidence of side-effects such as nausea, vomiting and hypotension during dialysis with large surface area dialysers was significantly lower when bicarbonate rather than an acetate dialysis fluid was used for the same degree of ultrafiltration. Since then, several manufacturers have produced bicarbonate proportionating machines but their use in the UK is still very limited.

11.4.3   Sequential ultrafiltration dialysis

The demonstration by Bergstrom *et al.* (1976) that fluid could be removed from overloaded uraemic patients by ultrafiltration without concomitant dialysis, with no change in blood pressure, pulse or plasma osmolality, despite a fall of up to 20% in plasma volume, aroused much interest in the dialysis field. At that time it was felt that lack of changes in plasma osmolality were responsible for the vascular stability but other groups, including our own (Walls *et al.*, 1979), have demonstrated that there is a rapid refilling of the intravascular space, both during and following such ultrafiltration. In addition, the refilling rate is proportional to the ultrafiltration rate and relates to changes in plasma oncotic pressure. This technique is now widely used, especially in dialysis patients with severe fluid overload where 2–3 l of fluid need to be removed within a short time. It has the advantage of being simple to perform using standard large surface area dialysers, in which it is possible to increase the hydrostatic pressure to 250–300 mmHg in the blood compartment.

The exact mechanism for the symptomatic hypotension or vascular instability seen during conventional haemodialysis is as yet not fully understood. However, Baldamus *et al.* (1980) have demonstrated that during haemofiltration and ultrafiltration without solute removal, there is an increase in both total peripheral resistance and sympathetic activity as measured by plasma noradrenaline levels, suggesting a normal physiological response to volume depletion. However, in the same patients during acetate haemodialysis there was no increase in sympathetic activity and a fall in total peripheral resistance. Similar findings were obtained during bicarbonate haemodialysis, although in this case there was a slight increase in total peripheral resistance. These results suggest that the presence of an autonomic neuropathy in uraemic patients is not a major factor responsible for vascular instability but that haemodialysis, especially with acetate dialysate, in some way interferes with the sympathetic regulation of total peripheral resistance.

11.4.4 Variable dialysis fluid sodium concentration

There is some evidence to suggest that increased sodium concentration in dialysis fluid may prevent or reduce the incidence of symptomatic hypotension (Van Stone and Cook, 1978) and this work needs further evaluation.

11.4.5 Clearance of substances of low molecular weight

Whilst the trend to shorten dialysis schedules has created problems in terms of symptomatic hypotension, little attention has been given to the removal of small molecular weight substances, such as urea, creatinine and uric acid, partly in the belief that they were 'non-toxic'. A recent important study from the USA has challenged this concept. This work, from the National Co-operative Dialysis Study (Lowrie *et al.*, 1981) summarizes the morbidity in 151 patients in a co-operative trial designed to evaluate the clinical effects of different dialysis prescriptions. The two variables in the four groups of patients studied were blood urea and dialysis time. The results demonstrate that patients with lower averaged blood urea (which takes into account both pre- and post-dialysis values) had significantly lower morbidity in terms of removal from the trial or hospitalization, provided that their protein intakes were adequate. There were no major correlations with the duration of dialysis or other factors concerned. The study group therefore recommend that a dialysis clearance-time combination, should be selected for the dialysis patient with an adequate protein intake to maintain his or her blood urea in the lower range, i.e. 18–20 mmol/l.

In summary, haemodialysis remains the cornerstone of the treatment of end-stage renal disease in the UK. Regrettably, not only has the UK fallen behind in terms of the number of patients accepted for treatment but also in developing and exploring the newer techniques in the haemodialysis field. The reason for this deficit is multifactorial and includes excessive workloads in individual renal units, a shortage of doctors committed to haemodialysis and a limited number of dialysis-orientated research workers. All of these depend predominantly on the lack of adequate financial assistance. These problems and many others associated with the treatment of end-stage renal disease have recently been reviewed and highlighted by Knapp (1982).

References

Alfrey, A.C., Le Gendre, G.R. and Kaehny, W.D. (1976). The dialysis encephalopathy syndrome: possible aluminium intoxication. *N. Engl. J. Med.*, **294**, 184

Baldamus, C.A., Ernst, W., Fassbinder, W. and Koch, K.M. (1980). Differing haemodynamic stability due to differing sympathetic response: comparison of ultrafiltration, haemodialysis and haemofiltration. *Proc. Eur. Dial. Transplant Assoc.*, **17**, 205

Bergström, J., Asaba, H., Fürst, P. and Oulès, R. (1976). Dialysis ultrafiltration and blood pressure. *Proc. Eur. Dial. Transplant Assoc.*, **13**, 293

Brynger, H., Brunner, F.P., Chantler, C., Donckerwolcke, R.A., Jacobs, C., Kramer, P., Selwood, N.H. and Wing, A.J. (1980). Combined report on regular dialysis and transplantation in Europe, X, 1979. *Proc. Eur. Dial. Transplant Assoc.*, **17**, 25

Cambi, V., Savazzi, G., Arisi, L., Bignardi, L., Bruschi, G., Rossi, E. and Migone, L. (1974). Short dialysis schedules (SDS) – finally ready to become a routine. *Proc. Eur. Dial. Transplant Assoc.*, **1**, 112

Dombey, S.L., Sagar, D. and Knapp, M.S. (1975). Chronic renal failure in Nottingham and requirements for dialysis and transplantation. *Br. Med. J.*, **1**, 484

Dunnill, M.S., Millard, P.R. and Oliver, D. (1977). Acquired cystic disease of the kidneys: a hazard of longterm intermittent maintenance haemodialysis. *J. Clin. Pathol.*, **30**, 868

Flendrig, J.A., Kruis, H. and Das, H.A. (1976). Aluminium intoxication: the cause of dialysis dementia. *Proc. Eur. Dial. Transplant Assoc.*, **13**, 355

Graefe, U., Milutinovich, J., Follette, W.C., Babb, A.L. and Scribner, B.H. (1977). Improved tolerance to rapid ultrafiltration with the use of bicarbonate in dialysate. *Proc. Eur. Dial. Transplant Assoc.*, **14**, 153

Henderson, L.W.A., Besorah, A., Michaels, A. and Bluemle, L.K.W. (1967). Blood purification by ultrafiltration and fluid replacement (diafiltration). *Trans. Am. Soc. Artif. Intern. Organs*, **13**, 216

Herr, H.W., Engen, D.E. and Hostetter, J. (1979). Malignancy in uremia: dialysis versus transplantation. *J. Urol.*, **121**, 584

Hodge, K.C., Day, J.P., O'Hara, M., Ackrill, P. and Ralston, A.J. (1981). Critical concentrations of aluminium in water used for dialysis. *Lancet*, **3**, 802

Knapp, M.S. (1982). Renal failure – dilemmas and developments. *Br. Med. J.*, **284**, 847

Laing, W. (1980). End-stage renal failure. *Office of Health Economics briefing* **No. 11**

Lowrie, E.G., Laird, N.M. Parker, T.F. and Sargent, J.A. (1981). Effect of the hemodialysis prescription on patient morbidity. *N. Engl. J. Med.*, **305**, 1176

Matas, A.J., Simmonds, R.L., Kjellstrand, C.M., Busselmeier, T.J. and Najavrian, J.S. (1975). Increased incidence of malignancy during chronic renal failure. *Lancet*, **1**, 883

Miach, P. J., Dawborn, J. K. and Xippel, J. (1976). Neoplasia in patients with chronic renal failure on long term dialysis. *Clin. Nephrol.,* **5,** 101

Parkinson, I. S., Ward, M. K., Feest, T. G., Fawcett, R. W. P. and Kerr, D. N. S. (1979). Fracturing dialysis osteodystrophy and dialysis encephalopathy: an epidemiological study. *Lancet,* **1,** 406

Platts, M. M., Goode, G. C. and Hislop, J. S. (1977). Composition of the domestic water supply and the incidence of fractures and encephalopathy in patients on home dialysis. *Br. Med. J.,* **2,** 657

Posen, G. A., Gray, D. G., Jaworski, Z. F., Couture, R. and Rashid, A. (1972). Comparison of renal osteodystrophy in patients dialyzed with deionised and non-deionised water. *Trans. Am. Soc. Artif. Intern. Organs,* **18,** 405

Quellhorst, E., Schueneman, B. and Boryhardt, J. (1978). Clinical and technical aspects of hemofiltration. *Artif. Organs,* **2,** 334

Shaldon, S. (1981). Progress in dialysis and the problems of patient tolerance to treatment. Zurukzoglu, W., Papadimitriou, M., Pyrpasopoulus, M., Sion, M. and Zamboulis, C. (eds.). *Proc. 8th Int. Cong. Nephrol.,* p. 689 (Basel: Karger)

Schneider, H., Streicher, E., Hachmann, H., Chmeil, H. and von Mylivs, U. (1977). Clinical experience with haemofiltration. *Proc. Eur. Dial. Transplant Assoc.,* **14,** 136

Sutherland, G. A., Glass, J. and Gabriel, R. (1977). Increased incidence of malignancy in renal failure. *Nephron,* **18,** 182

Uldall, P. R., Dyck, R. F., Woods, F., Merchant, N., Martin, G. S., Cardella, C. J., Sutton, D. and de Veber, G. A. (1979). A subclavian cannula for temporary vascular access for hemodialysis or plasmapheresis. *Dial. Transpl.,* **8,** 963

Van Stone, J. C. and Cook, J. (1978). Decreased post dialysis fatigue with increased dialysate sodium concentration. *Proc. Clin. Dial. Transplant Forum,* **8,** 152

Walls, J., Williams, P. F. and Byrom, N. P. (1979). Plasma volume changes in sequential ultrafiltration dialysis. UK Symposium: alternatives to haemo-dialysis. (London: Cordis Dow)

Walls, J. (1982). Disseminated malignancy from a primary growth in an end-stage kidney (In preparation)

Ward, M. K., Feest, T. G., Ellis, H. A., Parkinson, I. S. and Kerr, D. N. S. (1978). Osteomalacic dialysis osteodystrophy: evidence for a water-borne aetiological agent, probably aluminium. *Lancet,* **1,** 841

Wing, A. J. (1982). CAPD patients run greater risk of infection. *Nursing Mirror,* **154** (No. 12), 8

12

Continuous ambulatory peritoneal dialysis (CAPD) – current state in the United Kingdom
R. Gokal

12.1   INTRODUCTION

CAPD has gained increasing acceptance in the United Kingdom (UK) as a primary form of dialysis treatment for patients in end-stage renal failure (ESRF). The rate of increase in the number of patients on this treatment since 1979 has exceeded that of haemodialysis and of renal transplantation (Kerr, 1981). There is no doubt that CAPD provides an adequate form of dialysis treatment with a number of distinct advantages over haemodialysis. However, it does suffer from a few major problems which limit its use (Gokal *et al.*, 1980a; Nolph *et al.*, 1980). This paper outlines the current state of CAPD in the UK, together with the implications for the care of ESRF patients that arise from the rapid increase in the use of this technique.

12.2   CAPD IN THE UNITED KINGDOM

Because of strong economic reasons and the desire to place patients at home, renal transplantation and home haemodialysis have been the treatments of choice for renal replacement in the UK. The limitations imposed by this policy have meant that only half the expected number of new patients with ESRF have received dialysis treatment (expected rate of

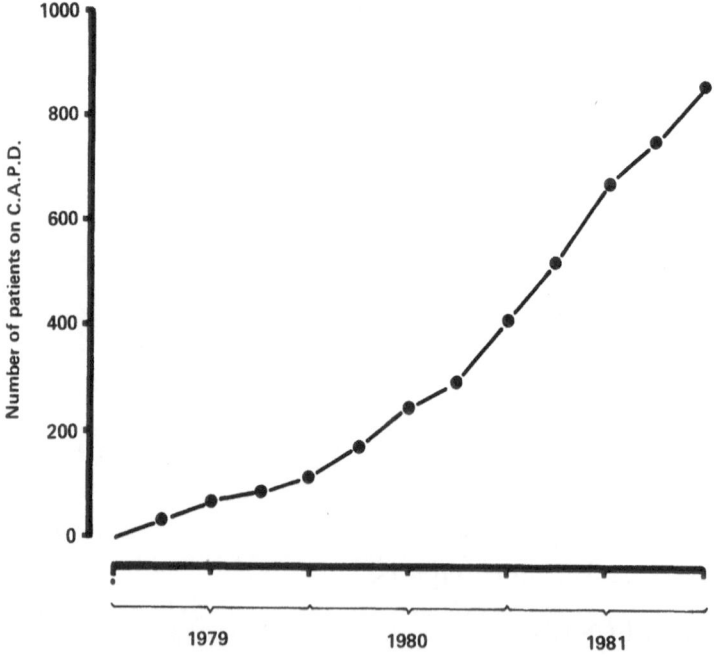

Figure 12.1   Expansion of CAPD in the United Kingdom over the 3 year period 1979–1981
The data were kindly provided by Travenol

new patients: 40 per million of population per year, aged 15 to 60, without systemic disease such as diabetes mellitus). Inadequate hospital haemodialysis facilities have meant that patients in the older age group (greater than 45 years) have been treated in much smaller numbers than in other European countries which currently have 55 'stations' per million of population as opposed to a figure of ten in the UK (Jacobs et al., 1981).

With the advent of CAPD in 1979, this picture changed in a way which has gathered momentum in the last 18 months. The rate of increase in the number of patients on CAPD has been dramatic and currently there are about 1000 patients receiving dialysis treatment by this technique representing 20% of the total dialysis population (Figure 12.1). The conditions that have favoured the deployment of this treatment in the UK are shown in Table 12.1. An important reason is the lack of in-centre haemodialysis facilities. However, this headlong rush into CAPD by nearly all the units (51 of the 55 UK units are using this technique) has had its problems. The EDTA data, based on a study of 330 patients show that the actuarial survival of patients on CAPD in the UK was about 80% at two years in 1980. However, the actuarial survival rate for the technique (including patients successfully transplanted) was 65% at one year and 40% at two years. When technique failure and death rate are combined, 50% of patients dropped out of CAPD at 1 year. Peritonitis was the commonest cause of failure in this group (Wing et al., 1981).

However, in units which have a wider and longer experience with the CAPD technique the drop-out rate is considerably better. Over the 3-year period since CAPD was introduced in Newcastle-upon-Tyne, the actuarial patient survival rate was 95% at two years, while the actuarial technique survival at two years, was 63% (Gokal et al., 1982a). Similarly, the drop-out and death rates in the six units with wide experience of CAPD in the UK (Table 12.2) show similar results with a total drop-out over 3 years of 25%,

Table 12.1 Conditions in the United Kingdom favouring the expansion of CAPD

Conditions related to other forms of therapy	
Transplantation	– shortage of donors
Hospital HD	– no building programme 10 'stations'/million of population (55 in W. Europe)
Minimal care	– ⟨ 1 unit/5 000 000
Home HD	– no increase in acceptance rate despite little financial restraint
Conditions related to CAPD	
No direct Government restriction on readmissions; PD fluid and equipment	
Modest outlay for staff and space	
Wide patient acceptance	
Short training time	

Table 12.2 Details of the number of patients treated with CAPD over the years 1978–82in six renal units in the UK, with associated failure data and peritonitis rates

Unit	Patients treated	Drop-outs	Failures			Peritonitis rate (episodes/patient week)
			Deaths			
			Peritonitis	Other	Peritonitis	
1	122	33	0	2	10	1 in 40
2	98	24	2	9	7	1 in 70
3	83	28	1	1	11	1 in 34
4	75	10	3	3	2	1 in 52
5	67	10	2	5	7	1 in 24
6	51	14	1	0	7	1 in 36
Total	496	119	9	20	53	
		24%			11%	

although actuarial data are not available. All the six units have a special training area and a planned training programme together with one or more nurses allocated specifically for CAPD training and management. Although these results are inferior to those of a home haemodialysis programme, the two populations of CAPD and home haemodialysis patients are likely to be different because of the patient selection policy and also because experience and expertise with haemodialysis are much greater. There are, as yet, no controlled comparative data on technique and patient survival on haemo-dialysis and CAPD. However, Mion (1982) in Montpellier, France, reports a 90% 7-year patient and technique survival on haemodialysis whereas the corresponding figure for his home CAPD programme in an equivalent age population of 15–55 years (excluding patients with additional risk factors) is 70% at 3 years.

What are the various reasons for this high drop-out rate in the UK? Undoubtedly some centres have undertaken this treatment without ade-quate facilities such as an area for CAPD, nursing staff, extra beds and haemodialysis back-up facilities for readmissions. These early problems add to the poor results reported. It is dangerous to regard CAPD as a procedure that can be undertaken as a 'one off' treatment or to commence a large pro-gramme without a training schedule, adequate facilities and staff to conduct it. These results may reflect an early 'learning' phase when 'teething' problems are overcome. It may be pertinent to know that although there is a genuine desire on the part of the centres in the UK to provide adequate facilities, financial restriction and, occasionally, obstinate Health Authori-ties make additional nursing and medical appointments extremely difficult and tiresome. There has to be a major change in policy at government level. The position is simply one of treating more patients; if this is desirable, then money and facilities must be made available. No doubt CAPD will provide a means whereby this is partly achieved; however, if CAPD is going to be used exclusively to increase the patient acceptance rate, thereby subjecting patients to this treatment who are better suited to in-centre (hospital) haemodialysis, the failure rate is likely to be high, thus increasing the strain on other hospital and haemodialysis resources and facilities.

12.3 REQUIREMENTS FOR A CAPD PROGRAMME

It is generally felt that undertaking CAPD in conditions not favourable to the technique produces bad results (Oreopoulos, 1979a; Gokal *et al.,* 1980a). Essential requirements in terms of area for CAPD, nursing and medical staff are outlined in Table 12.3. It is becoming apparent that because of the high fall-out rate in the UK and the high readmission rate for various complications (in Newcastle-upon-Tyne this was 11 days per patient year of treatment in the 3rd year of the programme, while a similar figure for Manchester in the first year was 25 days/patient year), back-up beds and short-term haemodialysis facilities are highly desirable. In addition, it is necessary to have an increase in the in-centre haemodialysis facilities to accommodate those who have failed with the CAPD technique.

In terms of the nursing staff requirement, it is essential to have, in overall charge, a nurse who does predominantly CAPD work (Oreopoulos, 1979a; Nolph, 1980). Other nurses can be co-opted under her as the programme enlarges. These nurses can be rotated through the haemodialysis and transplant nursing areas so as to alleviate the 'boredom' that may result from being associated with this single renal replacement procedure. No doubt the eventual make-up of the CAPD programme will be dependent upon local restrictions and circumstances. An ideal situation would be to blend CAPD into the existing renal replacement programme. In large programmes it may be desirable to have a home CAPD sister.

Table 12.3   Essential requirements of a CAPD programme

Nurses:	One sister in charge; about one additional nurse for every 15–20 patients
	Home CAPD sister for large programmes
	Integration/rotation of nurses through HD/TP
Area:	One to two 'beds' for training; area for set changes and OP
Back-up beds:	In ward – two to four beds for readmissions (one per 15–20 patients)
	HD – one to two stations for temporary haemodialysis and an increase in maintenance beds to accommodate 'drop-outs' from CAPD

12.4 PATIENT SELECTION FOR CAPD

It would appear that in the UK CAPD is utilized more often than not in patients who are either awaiting a place on a home haemodialysis training programme or who are unable to receive hospital haemodialysis. It has been considered that CAPD is indicated in the presence of cardiovascular instability, problems of vascular access and hypotension on haemodialysis, old age, diabetes mellitus and in patients living alone rather than as a primary form of therapy for ESRF. If selection is made in this way then the higher risk patients will be in the CAPD group with an associated increase in mortality and morbidity. In Newcastle-upon-Tyne in the first three years of an integrated dialysis and transplant programme, CAPD was used as a primary form of therapy in 54% of 173 new patients entering the programme. Here the technique survival results are comparable to those of other centres conducting CAPD (Gokal, 1982a; Mion, 1982).

As yet it is difficult to define the exact criteria for selection of a patient for CAPD. Most patients deemed suitable for independent haemodialysis at home would be equally suitable for CAPD. However, the profile of the patient prone to repeated peritonitis has not been established. Selection of the form of dialysis treatment for a patient who is equally suitable for home haemodialysis or CAPD is difficult. This will partly depend on patient preference, his social and work circumstances and perhaps transplantation prospects (Kerr, 1981). In patients with the rarer tissue types, in whom the chance of a quick transplant is small, home haemodialysis might be undertaken, whereas others could be placed on CAPD.

12.5 INTEGRATION OF CAPD WITH HAEMODIALYSIS

At the Manchester Royal Infirmary, England, an integrated dialysis and transplant programme exists. A new patient is assessed as being in an independent or dependent category based upon criteria such as intelligence, social standing, cleanliness and hygiene, ability to communicate and understanding of disease and technique (Figure 12.2). Patients designated as independent dialysis candidates are then assigned either to home/minimal care haemodialysis or to CAPD. The choice partly depends upon the availability of spaces for home haemodialysis training, patient preference, and medical indications. However, currently some patients who are deemed suitable only for dependent dialysis are being tried out on CAPD because of the lack of in-centre haemodialysis facilities. The aim is, nevertheless, to try and tailor the treatment to the patient's medical and social needs. In this integrated programme, interchange of therapy can take place, with transplantation as the eventual goal. If more kidney grafts become available and the waiting time for transplantation is reduced considerably, then the treatment of choice would appear to be CAPD. However, there is a danger that patients

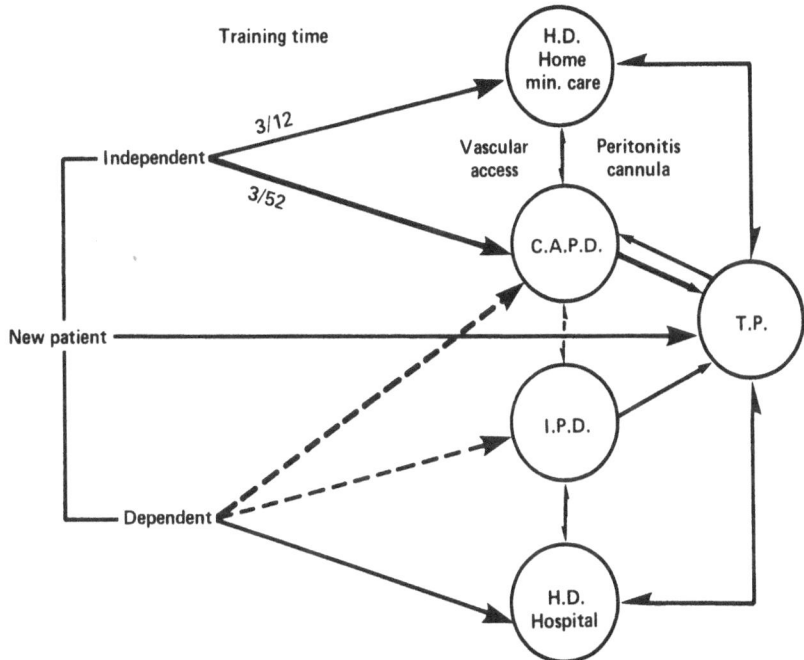

Figure 12.2 Schematic representation of the integrated dialysis and transplant programme as practised at the Manchester Royal Infirmary. The bold dotted line indicates placement onto CAPD of 'dependent' patients who would be more suited to hospital haemodialysis but who are unable to receive this because of the lack of adequate HD facilities

min care = minimal care, IPD = intermittent peritoneal dialysis, TP = transplantation, HD = haemodialysis

suitable for transplantation would receive the grafts, leaving a core of high risk patients on CAPD or haemodialysis.

As yet it is difficult to assess the exact role that CAPD will play in renal replacement therapy. Its longterm future is still unknown. It is unlikely to supersede haemodialysis as a primary form of dialysis therapy, but in any integrated programme, anything up to a quarter of the patients are likely to be managed by CAPD.

12.6 ADVANTAGES OF CAPD

These are outlined in Table 12.4. There is no doubt that the patients feel very well, something that is most noticeable in patients transferred from haemodialysis therapy. These patients enjoy the freedom from the machine, the liberal fluid and dietary allowances and the freedom of travel.

The biochemical control is good with adequate steady state values for plasma urea and creatinine concentrations. Plasma sodium, potassium and bicarbonate concentrations, are also maintained within normal limits on a free diet (Gokal *et al.*, 1980a). In addition, there is a better clearance of

Table 12.4   Advantages and disadvantages of CAPD

Advantages

(1) Patient well being; increased diet, fluid, and travel freedom

(2) Good steady state biochemical control

(3) Improved control of anaemia,
                     hypertension
                     and bone disease

(4) Treatment feasible in children,
                     elderly
                     and diabetes mellitus

(5) Short training time, wide patient acceptance

(6) Cheaper than haemodialysis

Disadvantages

(1) High peritonitis rate and high technique failure rate

(2) Mechanical problems with PD catheters, connectors and lines

(3) Gastrointestinal problems – hernias

(4) Patient 'dislikes' with time
       – no free days 'chore',
       – worry of peritonitis,
       – up to 3 hours/day,
       – disfigurement

(5) Obesity and hyperlipidaemia
       ? malnutrition

(6) Loss of ultrafiltration and peritoneal clearances

'middle molecules' (five times that achieved on 15 hours haemodialysis per week) (Oreopoulos *et al.*, 1979b) and this may be part of the reason for the increased well-being. The latter may also be related to the rise in haemoglobin which is seen in most patients on CAPD and which reaches a plateau at a mean level of about 10 g/dl (Gokal *et al.*, 1980a, Nolph *et al.*, 1980). This increase is most dramatic in the first 6 months when it is related to haemoconcentration resulting from the better ultrafiltration achieved on CAPD. The continued increase in the haemoglobin levels thereafter is secondary to a true rise in the red cell mass (de Paepe *et al.*, 1981).

The ease of ultrafiltration and sodium removal allows better control of hypertension. Hypotensive episodes noted in the earlier reports were probably related to over-zealous ultrafiltration and sodium loss and the use of a sodium concentration of 130 mmol/l in the dialysis fluid (Oreopoulos, 1979b).

The easier control of plasma phosphate is generally reported in CAPD patients with much less necessity for the use of oral phosphate binding agents. Plasma calcium levels are returned to normal with treatment (Gokal *et al.*, 1980b). In conjunction with this, parathyroid hormone (PTH) levels decrease, probably as a result of the clearance of PTH in the dialysate (Delmez *et al.*, 1980). In addition, there is a loss of 25-hydroxycholecalciferol into the dialysate leading to low plasma levels (Gokal *et al.*, 1982b). Overall, it appears that patients on CAPD need calcium supplements (calcium carbonate 1–3 g daily) and cautious vitamin D replacement. Based on this regimen there has been good control of histological renal osteodystrophy although some centres do report radiological deterioration (Calderaro *et al.*, 1980).

In Newcastle-upon-Tyne the histological evidence of renal osteodystrophy improved significantly in studies of 30 paired bone biopsies done one year apart, with a further nine studied at 2 years. It remains to be seen whether this improved control of renal osteodystrophy in the early years is maintained with prolonged CAPD.

Another advantage of this treatment is that it can be used in children, the elderly and in patients with diabetes mellitus. In the diabetic group, the use of intraperitoneal insulin has been shown to give good control of blood sugar with stabilization or even improvement in retinopathy (Mion, 1982; Flynn, 1980).

12.7 DISADVANTAGES OF CAPD

12.7.1 Peritonitis

This complication is one of the major drawbacks to this otherwise simple and relatively convenient method of dialysis treatment. It is still a common cause of technical failure. In the Newcastle-upon-Tyne centre, of the 33 patient failures on CAPD (out of a total of 122 patients who received this treatment) 19 were related to peritonitis. These patients were transferred to maintenance haemodialysis. In four patients there was total obliteration of the peritoneal cavity with adhesions following pseudomonas peritonitis. The drop-out rates related to peritonitis and deaths from peritonitis in the six units in the country are shown in Table 12.2. Overall, the peritonitis rate reported in most centres with extensive experience is one episode per patient year. Therefore, with the current techniques and staff and facilities available, it is unlikely that one is going to be able to do very much better. However, the use of in-line filters has reduced the infection rate in France (Mion *et al.*, 1981) and further improvements in the incidence of peritonitis can only come about with a new generation of connectors, lines and catheters, peritoneal dialysis fluids and a better understanding of the pathophysiology and treatment of peritonitis.

Peritonitis is almost invariably related to a break in the sterile technique, fluid leaks from catheters and exit site, and exit site infections; this is reflected in the fact that more than half the episodes are due to skin organisms. However, bacteria can get across the colon and this occurs more frequently in patients with diverticular disease. Prevention of peritonitis depends very much upon developing connectors and systems which do not depend upon the ability of the patient to perform a sterile exchange procedure. The introduction of the luer lock connectors and new connector developments using ultra violet light, should minimize the infection risk, especially if these are used in conjunction with an in-line filter. However, the role of the nursing staff and the use of a special area for training and set changes is of vital importance in controlling the infection rate. Several studies have shown that when CAPD is conducted in areas unsuited for the technique, or performed with inadequate nursing staff, the peritonitis rate increases dramatically (Gokal *et al.*, 1980a).

Currently there is still uncertainty about the treatment of peritonitis. It is widely held that the best route of administration of antibiotic treatment is via the peritoneum. This is based on the desire to establish a high concentration of antibiotics at the site of the infection. A broad spectrum antibiotic, usually a cephalosporin, is used blindly as a first line antibiotic and many centres in the UK use cefuroxime in a dose of 200 mg/l. CAPD is usually continued after an initial lavage if the patient is very toxic (Vas *et al.*, 1981). However, the duration of therapy and the route of subsequent therapy after the initial period is still not well defined. Since half the infections are caused by skin organisms, it is felt that gram-positive infections should be treated for 5–7 days with the appropriate anti-biotics, while gram-negative organisms, which are more prone to abscess formation and scarring within the peritoneum, need longer treatment. Adequate therapy obviously depends upon isolation of the causative organism and many centres report that up to 20% of episodes of peritonitis are culture negative. This may be a reflection of the culture techniques and close liaison with the bacteriological department is essential for good management of CAPD peritonitis.

Treatment whenever possible should be undertaken at home. This minimizes hospitalization. In Newcastle-upon-Tyne in 1981 48% of the episodes were managed entirely at home while a further 36% of patients spent only the initial few days in hospital with subsequent management at home. A number of other problems still persist and require close investigation. There are problems of exit site infection and the use of single or double cuff Tenckhoff catheters. Nor is it clear whether a dressing is necessary over the exit site.

The use of cumulative treatment periods to express incidence rates can be misleading when the population is large and individual treatment times are short relative to the calculated incidence interval. There is also a need to obtain a statistically valid method of comparing infection rates, and thereby evaluate technique modifications and assess the efficiency of new techniques. For these reasons a life table method of actuarial analysis is now very much the preferred method of expressing the incidence of peritonitis. Each peritonitis episode is considered as a 'death' event for computing the actuarial curve. The results are expressed as the percentage risk of having a peritonitis episode (Randerson and Farrell, 1981a). Based on this method the actuarial risk of patients having a first episode of peritonitis is 50% at 12 months which is equivalent to an incidence of one episode for every 19 patient-months of treatment (Mion *et al.*, 1982).

12.7.2 Hospitalization

One of the major worries related to the use of CAPD has been the high rate of readmissions, averaging between 15–25 days per patient year (Nolph, see Chapter 7). Peritonitis is still the commonest cause for admission but mechannical problems related to catheters and medical problems in the elderly are other important reasons. In the Newcastle-upon-Tyne renal unit, readmissions in 1981 amounted to a mean of 11 days per patient-year of which 4.2 days were secondary to peritonitis, 3.0 for mechancial problems and the remainder for other reasons. In Manchester, in the first year of CAPD, part of which was in conditions not suited for undertaking the technique, hospitalization was 26 days/patient year of which 14 were related to peritonitis. The Newcastle figure compares favourably with home haemodialysis readmission rates. Part of this improvement is related to the policy in Newcastle-upon-Tyne of treating as many patients as possible at home when they have episodes of peritonitis. The number of episodes treated at home increased from 0 in 1979 to 48% in 1981.

12.7.3 Obesity and hyperlipidaemia

A large number of patients gain weight and this may well be related initially to increased appetite and calorie intake derived from the absorption of dextrose from the peritoneal fluid. The initial weight gain may well reflect some 'catching up' but in some patients substantial weight increases have been noted of up to 30% of their starting weight (Gokal *et al.*, 1982b). In a few patients the increase in weight may not necessarily reflect a better nutritional status. The protein intake can diminish by up to 20% of that which is recommended (Baeyer *et al.*, 1981). The hypertriglyceridaemia and hypercholesterolaemia may well be related to the increase in weight and to dextrose absorption; it seems to be more marked in those patients who are already hyperlipidaemic at the start of CAPD (Gokal *et al.*, 1981; Roncari *et al.*, 1982).

12.7.4 Loss of ultrafiltration

This has been reported in a small number of patients most of whom have had peritonitis as an underlying aetiology. However, Mion (1982) has reported patients who have had IPD and/or CAPD for prolonged periods of time, usually in excess of 2 years, in whom loss of ultrafiltration has not been related to peritonitis. This is obviously worrying as is the potential loss of peritoneal clearances with time (Randerson and Farrell, 1981b).

12.7.5   Other problems

These include inguinal, umbilical, incisional and diaphragmatic hernias (Ramos et al., 1982). A fair number of patients on longterm therapy do seem to tire and find the exchange procedure a 'chore'. The daily three to four exchanges leave little respite in some cases and this may lead to breaks in technique and peritonitis. Some patients live in fear and trepidation of peritonitis while others with drainage problems may well spend up to 3 hours a day doing exchanges.

12.8   FUTURE DEVELOPMENTS

The future of CAPD rests entirely upon the reduction of the peritonitis rate which in itself is dependent upon improvement in the connectors, lines and catheters. The physiology of peritonitis needs to be better understood. An exciting development is the use of 3 litre exchanges three times a day rather than the usual four × 2 litre exchanges (Twadki and Janicka, 1981). The increased volume is dependent upon the vital capacity and respiratory reserve of the patient. For those patients who can tolerate the 3 litre, there is increased ultra-filtration and better dialysis. Whether this increases the mechanical and hernia problems remains to be seen. The search for better osmotic agents continues and could lead to exciting developments. Aminoacids and dextrans have been tried. The ideal agent might lead to a decrease in the number of exchanges and hence of the peritonitis rate and minimize the metabolic complications.

12.9   CONCLUSION

CAPD is an exciting form of treatment. There are some distinct advantages over haemodialysis but it does suffer from serious complications, peritonitis being the most important. Currently the drop-out rate from the technique is very high in the UK and needs to be reduced quite dramatically before it becomes generally accepted as a primary form of dialysis treatment. None-theless, it is currently being used in about a fifth of all patients receiving dialysis treatment and it is likely that this will be the projected percentage in the future. Its better deployment will depend upon a lessening of the complication rate and an increase in the transplantation rate.

However, decreasing the complication rate depends upon how CAPD is used. It should be regarded as a primary form of dialysis treatment and its proper deployment depends on the enthusiasm of the consultant nephrologist and the unit towards CAPD. It should not be undertaken in isolation or as a one-off treatment procedure. In a programme of reasonable size success will depend on having an area reserved for CAPD, adequate nursing staff and back-up facilities. In addition, greater hospital haemodialysis back-up is required for those that drop out from CAPD or require temporary haemodialysis.

CAPD is an exciting treatment with tremendous potential. It is here to stay and we need to develop techniques and methods to minimize the complications. For the best results it should be utilized as a primary form of dialysis treatment in an integrated dialysis and transplantation programme.

12.10 ACKNOWLEDGEMENTS

The author wishes to thank the renal units in Newcastle-upon-Tyne, Oxford, Royal Free Hospital, London Hospital and Sheffield for data relating to their CAPD programmes; and the Newcastle renal unit for results of studies related to peritonitis and histological bone disease in CAPD patients.

References

Baeyer, H., Gahl, G. M., Riedinger, H., Borowzak, B. and Kessel, M. (1981). Unexpected alteration of nutritional habits in patients undergoing CAPD. In Gahl, G. M., Kessel, M. and Nolph, K. D. (eds.). *Advances in Peritoneal Dialysis*, pp. 408–12 (Amsterdam: Excerpta Medica)

Calderaro, V., Oreopoulos, D. G., Mesina, H. E., Ogilvie, R., Khanna, R., Quinton, C., Murray, T. and Carmichael, D. (1980). The evolution of renal osteodystrophy in patients undergoing CAPD. *Proc. Eur. Dial. Transplant Assoc.*, **17**, 533

Delmez, J., Slatopolsky, E., Gearing, B. and Harter, H. (1980). Effects of CAPD in PTH and calcium metabolism. *Abstract. Proc. Am. Soc. Nephrol.*, **13**, 38

Flynn, C. T. (1980). CAPD in diabetic patients. In Legrain, M. (ed.). *Continuous Ambulatory Peritoneal Dialysis*. pp. 187–193. (Amsterdam: Excerpta Medica)

Gokal, R., McHugh, M., Fryer, R., Ward, M. K. and Kerr, D. N. S. (1980a). CAPD: one year's experience in a UK dialysis unit. *Br. Med. J.*, **287**, 474

Gokal, R., Fryer, R., McHugh, M., Ward, M. K. and Kerr, D. N. S. (1980b). Calcium and phosphate control in CAPD. In Legrain, M., (eds.). *Continuous Ambulatory Peritoneal Dialysis*. pp. 283–291. (Amsterdam: Excerpta Medica)

Godal, R., Ramos, J., McHugh, J., Ward, M. K. and Kerr, D. N. S. (1981). Hyperlipidaemia in patients on CAPD. In Gahl, G. M., Kessel, M. and Nolph, K. D. (eds.). *Advances in Peritoneal Dialysis*. pp. 430–433. (Amsterdam: Excerpta Medica)

Gokal, R., Ramos, M. J., Ward, M. K., Wilkinson, R., Elliot, W., Ellis, H. A. and Kerr, D. M. S. (1982a). 3 years experience of CAPD in a UK dialysis unit. *Q. J. Med.* (submitted for publication)

Gokal, R., Ramos, J.M., Ellis, H.A., Parkinson, I., Sweetman, V., Dewar, J., Ward, M.K. and Kerr, D.N.S. (1982b). Histological renal osteodystrophy, 25 OHD$_3$ and aluminium levels in patients on CAPD. *Kidney Int.,* (In press)

Jacobs, C., Broyer, M., Brunner, F.P., Brynger, H., Donckerwolcke, R.A., Kramer, P., Selwood, N.H., Wing, A.J. and Blake, P.H. (1981). Combined report on regular dialysis and transplantation in Europe, 1980. *Proc. Eur. Dial. Transplant Assoc.,* **18,** 4

Kerr, D.N.S. (1981). Dialysis strategy: cost and effectiveness. *Proc. Eur. Dial. Transplant Assoc.,* **18, 664**

Mion, C., Slingeneyer, A. and Conaud, B. (1981). CAPD in France: results of a national survey and 2 years experience at one centre. In Atkins, R.C., Thomson, N. and Farrell, P.C. (eds.). *Peritoneal Dialysis.* pp. 126–135. (Edinburgh: Churchill Livingstone)

Mion, C., (1982). Experience with CAPD in France. Paper presented at *Second Spanish Symposium on CAPD,* March 1982. *Nefrologia* (In press)

Nolph, K., Sorkin, M., Rubin, J., Arfarra, D., Prowant, B., Fruto, L. and Kennedy, D. (1980). CAPD. Three years experience. *Ann. Int. Med.,* **92,** 7

Oreopoulos, D.G. (1979a) Requirements for the organisation of a CAPD programme. *Nephron,* **24,** 261

Oreopoulos, D.G., Robson, M., Faller, B., Ogilvie, R., Rappoport, A., DeVeber, G.A. (1979b). CAPD: a new era in the treatment of chronic renal failure. *Clin. Nephrol.,* **11, 125**

de Paepe, M., Lamiere, N., Schelstraete, K. and Kingoir, S. (1981). Changes in red cell mass, plasma volume and haematocrit in patients on CAPD. *Proc. Eur. Dial. Transplant Assoc.,* **18, 286**

Ramos, J.M., Burke, D.A. and Veitch, P.S. (1982). Hernia of Morgagni in patients on CAPD. *Lancet,* **1,** 162

Randerson, D.H. and Farrell, P.C. (1981a). Analysis of peritonitis data in CAPD. In Gahl, G.M., Kessel, M. and Nolph, K.D. (eds.). *Advances in Peritoneal Dialysis.* pp. 265–269. (Amsterdam: Excerpta Medica)

Randerson, D.H. and Farrell, P.C. (1981b). Long term peritoneal clearances in CAPD In Atkins, R.C., Thomson, N.M. and Farrell, P.C. (eds.). *Peritoneal Dialysis.* pp. 22–29. (Edinburgh: Churchill Livingstone)

Roncari, D.A.K., Breckenridge, W.C., Khanna, R. and Oreopoulos, D.G. (1982). Rise in HDL-Cholesterol in some patients with CAPD. *Peritoneal Dial. Bull.,* **1,** 136

Twadki, Z. and Janicka, L. (1981). Three exchanges with a 2.5l volume for CAPD. *Kidney Int.,* **20,** 281

Vas, S.I., Duwe, A. and Weatherhead, J. (1981). Natural defence mechanisms of the peritoneum: The effect of PD fluid on polymorphonuclear cells. In Atkins, R.C., Thomson, N. and Farrell, P.C. (eds.). *Peritoneal Dialysis.* pp. 41–51. (Edinburgh: Churchill Livingstone)

Wing, A.J., Broyer, M., Brunner, F.P., Brynger, H., Donckerwolcke, R.A., Jacobs, C., Kramer, P., Selwood, N.H. and Blake, P.H. (1981). Treatment of end stage renal failure in the United Kingdom EDTA Registry analysis. In Bradley, B and Moras, D. (eds.). *UK Transplant Service Review 1981.* pp. 71–94. South Western Regional Transfusion Centre, Southmead Road, Bristol, UK

13

Future developments in renal transplantation
R. F. M. Wood

13.1 INTRODUCTION

There have been some exciting advances in transplant research in the past 5 years which are now beginning to have an impact on clinical practice. In this chapter six topics have been selected which are likely to have a profound influence on the results of renal transplantation:

The centre effect,
Tissue typing,
Cytotoxic antibody testing,
Blood transfusion and allograft enhancement,
Immunosuppression and
Immunological monitoring.

13.2 THE CENTRE EFFECT

Significant differences in the results of transplantation between the individual units in Great Britain and Ireland first came to light in the UK Transplant Annual Report (1978/79). This 'Centre Effect' is illustrated in Figure 13.1, showing a scatter of graft survival at 1 year from over 80% in the best units to less than 40% in the centres with the poorest results. The financial implications alone are considerable as patients whose transplants fail usually have a prolonged period of hospitalization before eventually being returned to dialysis. In human terms the cost of graft failure is much higher; the patient will usually have been treated with large doses of immunosuppression to reverse rejection with a significant increase in the incidence of serious infection and death. In addition survival rates are

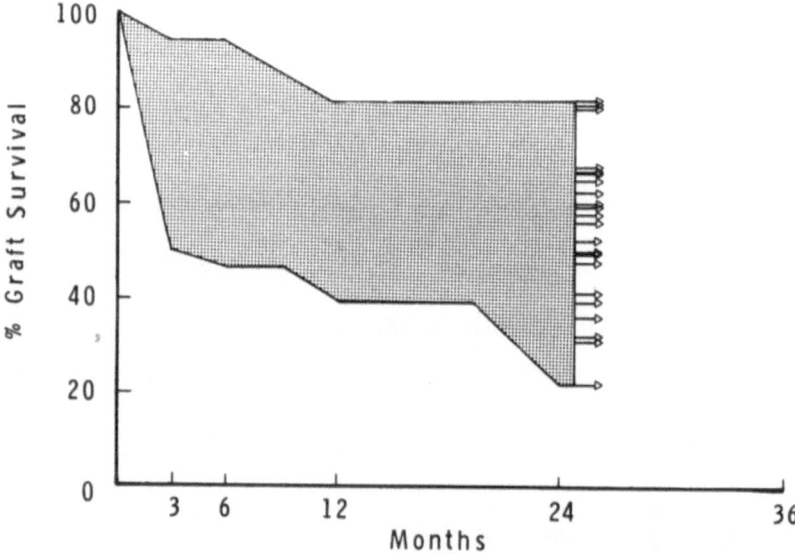

Figure 13.1 'The centre effect', the variation in graft survival between centres in the United Kingdom (reproduced by permission of the UK Transplant Service)

always best after first transplants and, due to sensitization, it may be extremely difficult to re-graft patients whose initial cadaver kidney has failed. For the future development of transplantation this must be one of the most important areas to which thought should be given. If the factors responsible for good graft survival in the best centres and those responsible for the adverse levels of graft survival in the poor centres could be identified, it might be possible to propose a scheme of selection and management which would greatly improve the overall results. The centre size is certainly one important factor and the statistics from the European Dialysis and Transplant Association (EDTA) for 1978–80 (Jacobs *et al.,* 1981) show that first cadaver graft survival at 1 year, in recipients between 15 and 45 years, was 70% in centres transplanting over 50 cases a year and only marginally less in centres performing 25–49 grafts per year. However, in units with a transplant rate of 10–24 cases per year the one year graft survival was only 60% and fell to 57% in units performing less than 10 operations per year. Therefore, although 'satellite' dialysis units may be a viable concept, transplantation should probably be concentrated in centres large enough to provide a full range of back-up facilities, including immunological expertise. Other reasons for the 'centre effect' are undoubtedly multifactorial, but there may be a number of relatively simple factors which are of particular importance.

The British Transplantation Society has taken up the challenge of investigating the 'centre effect' and is sending a team including a nephrologist, a surgeon and an immunologist to visit a selection of centres with both good and poor results. It is hoped that this study will provide guide lines for 'good practice' in transplantation which will help to prevent avoidable failures.

13.3   TISSUE TYPING

Snell (1948) coined the term 'histocompatibility antigens' to describe the determinants relevant to matching for transplantation between strains of 'in-bred' mice. An equivalent system in the human – the HLA system – was subsequently described by Payne (1964). The major histocompatibility complex in the human is located on the short arm of chromosome number six (Figure 13.2).

13.3.1   HLA-A and B locus matching

The originally described HLA-A and B loci have been used as the basis of tissue matching and organ sharing for the past 15 years. Tissue types are established serologically in a micro-lymphocytotoxity test. Some 20 different specifications have now been established at the A locus and over 30 at the B locus. Each individual has two A and two B locus determinants

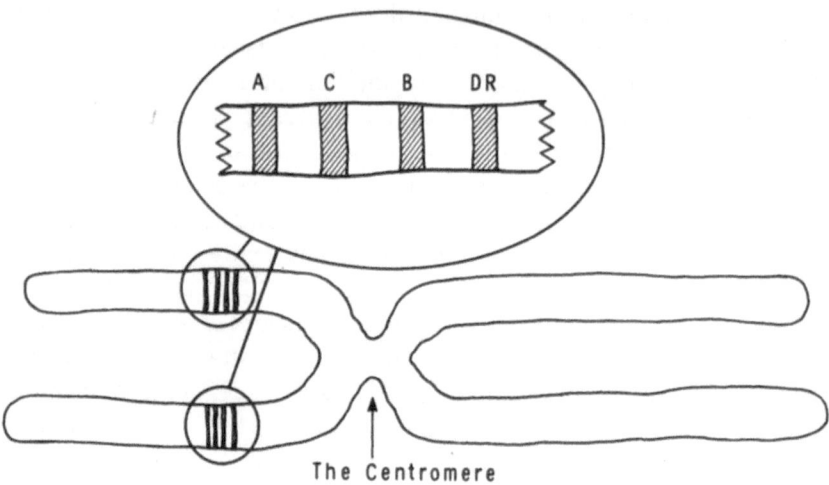

Figure 13.2 The human major histocompatibility complex, situated on the short arm of chromosome six. Showing the relationship of the HLA-A, B, C and DR loci

and there are therefore a vast number of possible different phenotypes. For many patients on the transplant waiting list there is virtually no hope of obtaining an identical kidney on the basis of A and B locus matching.

The value of HLA-A and B locus matching in transplantation remains controversial. The London Transplant Group reporting the results of 899 transplants performed between 1969 and 1979 show a highly significant influence of A and B matching on graft survival (Festenstein *et al.*, 1981). The importance of the B locus has been stressed by the Newcastle unit who have over 80% graft survival at 3 years in transfused patients who received a donor kidney identical at the B locus (Dewar *et al.*, 1982). However, the results from large collected series, such as the 2014 cases reported by Opelz and Terasaki (1982), have failed to show any correlation between graft survival and HLA-A and B locus matching. Figure 13.3 shows the statistics for the United Kingdom from the UK Transplant Annual Report (1978–79). Although the curves are appropriately stratified for match grade the differences in survival between 'well-matched' and 'poorly-matched' kidneys are small and disappear completely if the graphs are re-drawn to show failures from rejection alone. This may indicate that some poor results in mis-matched patients are due to urgent transplants in high-risk individuals.

13.3.2 D locus matching

The D locus, situated closer to the centromere of chromosome six (Figure 13.2), has been known to have an important influence on the outcome of transplantation. However, typing for the D locus could only be achieved by mixed lymphocyte culture over 5 days and was therefore only possible in live donor transplantation. The discovery of D locus antigens on the surface of B lymphocytes paved the way for a serological determination of D locus compatibility – DR matching (Bodmer *et al.*, 1978). Since there is a single DR locus, only two matches are required for complete identity. In addition, only ten specificities have so far been defined at the DR locus and, even if a few further determinants are discovered, matching for DR will remain relatively straightforward. The results of DR matching in Oxford are shown in Figure 13.4 with 78% one year graft survival in patients receiving DR identical kidneys. This was significantly better ($p = 0.02$) than the 62% one year survival in patients whose transplants were mis-matched for DR. Further information on the value of DR matching in large series is

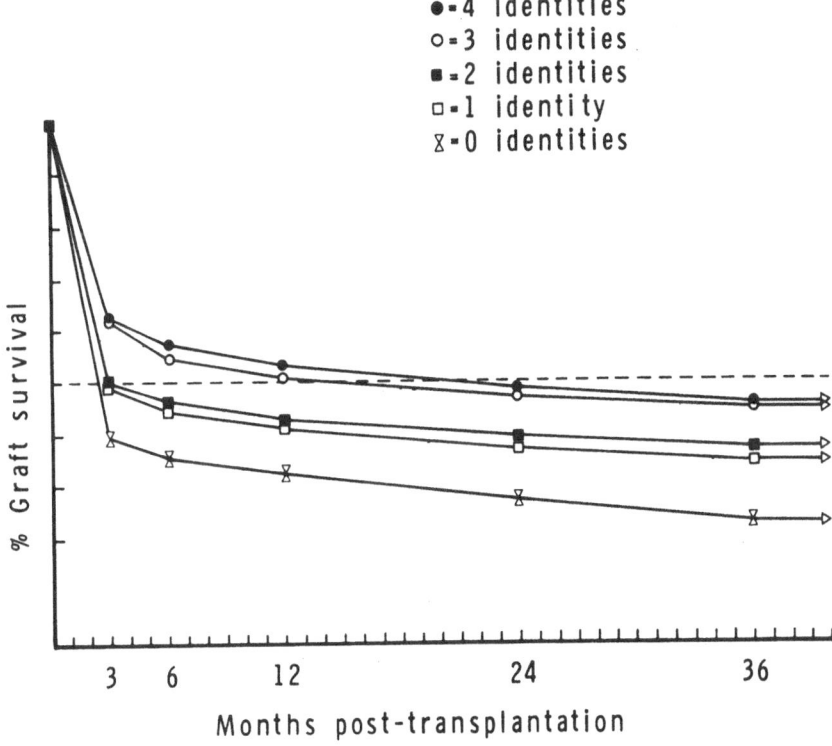

Figure 13.3 The effect of HLA-A and B locus matching on graft survival in the United Kingdom. Figures from the UK Transplant Service report for 1978-79 (reproduced by permission of the UK Transplant Service)

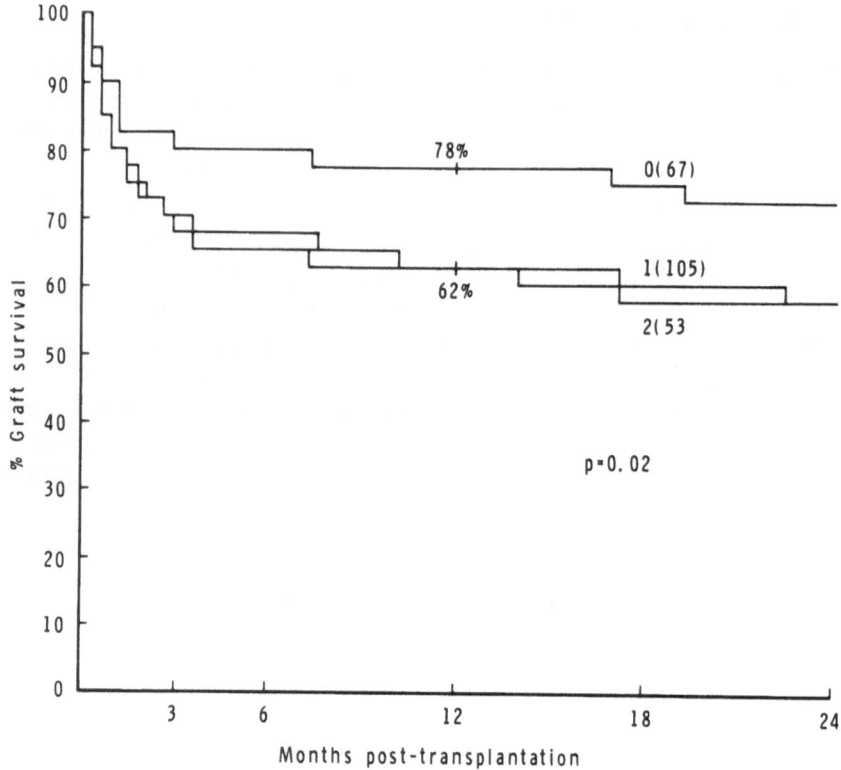

Figure 13.4   Results of DR matching in Oxford, showing a statistically significant benefit for patients receiving a DR identical kidney

still awaited. However, the pooled results from North America already show a statistically significant advantage for DR matched over DR mis-matched donor recipient combinations (Opelz and Terasaki, 1982).

Increasing knowledge of the major histocompatibility system will un-doubtedly be acquired during the next few years. In some ways this additional information may only complicate the practical problem of matching donors and recipients. However, for patients with a given tissue type it may be possible in future to identify specificities to which they will have a strong response and therefore be able to map out a series of 'acceptable' donor tissue-types for each individual recipient.

13.4   Cytotoxic antibody testing

Pre-formed cytotoxic antibodies, capable of causing hyperacute rejection, may be present in the sera of potential transplant recipients as a result of blood transfusion, pregnancy or a previous failed transplant. Hyperacute rejection is an irreversible process characterized by rapid destruction of the vascular endothelium within the graft, due to activation of both the complement and coagulation systems. Platelet thrombi form in the glomerular capillary loops, blocking the whole micro-circulation of the kidney. The detection of these antibodies by a pre-transplant cross-match test is therefore one of the routines of clinical transplantation and a positive response has been regarded as an absolute contraindication to operation. Antibodies occur much more frequently than was previously recognized and if serum samples are collected around the time of blood transfusion, at the time of acute rejection and after graft nephrectomy, there will frequently be significant levels of antibody activity when the sera are tested against a panel of normal lymphocytes (Morris and Ting, 1981). Routine screening for cytotoxic antibodies has revealed the presence of a sizeable group of patients with high levels of antibody who have been regarded as 'untransplantable' because of the risks of hyperacute rejection. However, the development of more sophisticated analyses of the cross-match test has demonstrated that not all these antibodies are liable to cause hyperacute rejection. The work of Ting (Ting and Morris, 1977 and 1978) has shown that many patients have auto-antibodies which, although causing a cytotoxic reaction with donor T and B lymphocytes *in vitro*, will not cause damage *in vivo*. The presence of these auto-antibodies can be detected by screening the sera of potential recipients against a panel of B lymphocytes from patients with chronic lymphatic leukaemia (CLL). These CLL cells express HLA-A, B and DR antigens on their surface and a positive reaction to CLL cells indicates the presence of a broadly reactive cytotoxic antibody within the serum. However, patients who have only auto-antibodies will not react with CLL cells. The results of transplantation in Oxford in patients with positive cross-matches due to auto-reactive antibodies are shown in Figure 13.5. There is no difference in graft survival between the patients who were cross-match negative and those who had either a positive B cell cross-match or a positive B + T cell cross-match due to auto-reactive antibodies.

Despite the satisfactory results of transplantation in patients with auto-antibodies there remains the problem of transplantation in patients with broadly reactive antibodies, cytotoxic for over 90% of panel lymphocytes. For these patients successful transplantation is only possible with a well-matched kidney, avoiding HLA identities to which the individual has previously been sensitized. One of the proposals from the UK Transplant Service is a tissue typing plate of serum samples from highly sensitized patients distributed to all the tissue-typing centres in the country. Cells from every cadaver donor would be tested using this plate in the hope of finding the highly sensitized patient a kidney with a realistic chance of success.

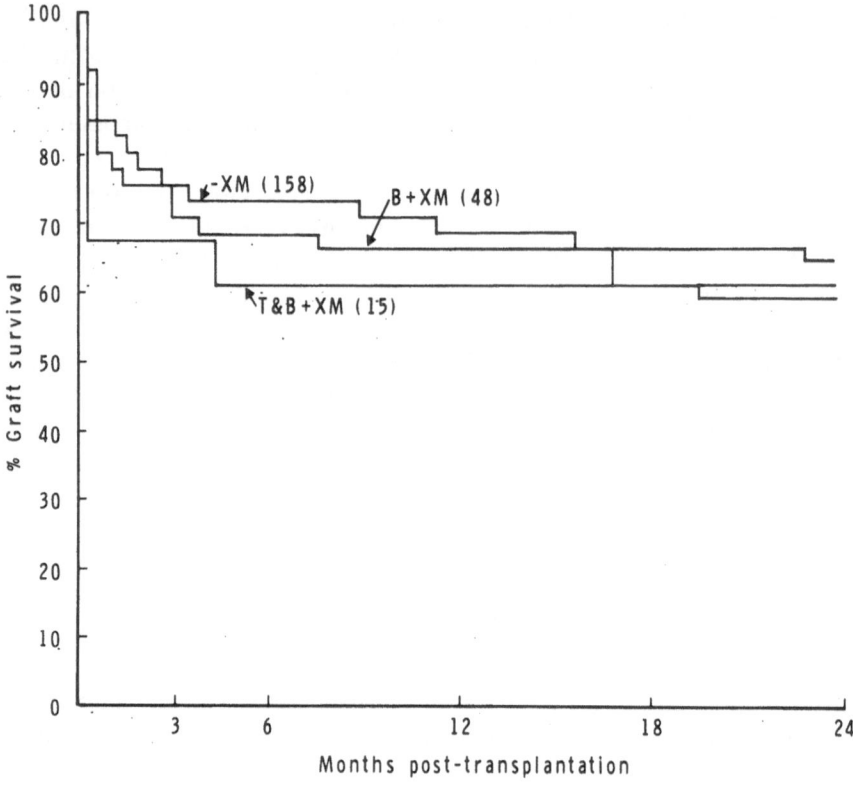

Figure 13.5   Graft survival in the Oxford series following transplantation in the face of a positive cross-match due to auto-reactive antibodies

13.5   Blood transfusion and allograft enhancement

During the 1960s the vast majority of patients receiving transplants had been polytransfused while on dialysis. It was recognized that transfusion caused an increased incidence of cytotoxic antibody formation and it was felt that transplant results would probably be better in non-sensitized patients who had never been transfused. Improved dialysis techniques and the risks of hepatitis led to a reduced incidence of blood transfusions in dialysis units and by the early 1970s there was a large pool of dialysis patients who had never been transfused. However, it soon became apparent that non-transfused patients faired relatively poorly after transplantation and that unplanned blood transfusion had a beneficial effect on allograft survival (Opelz *et al.*, 1973; van Es and Balner, 1979; Opelz and Terasaki, 1980). Experience in Oxford (Figure 13.6) has shown that one year graft survival after only one or two units of blood is significantly better, at 81%, than the 56% one year graft survival in non-transfused patients. Although many units now adopt a policy of deliberate transfusion, concern has been

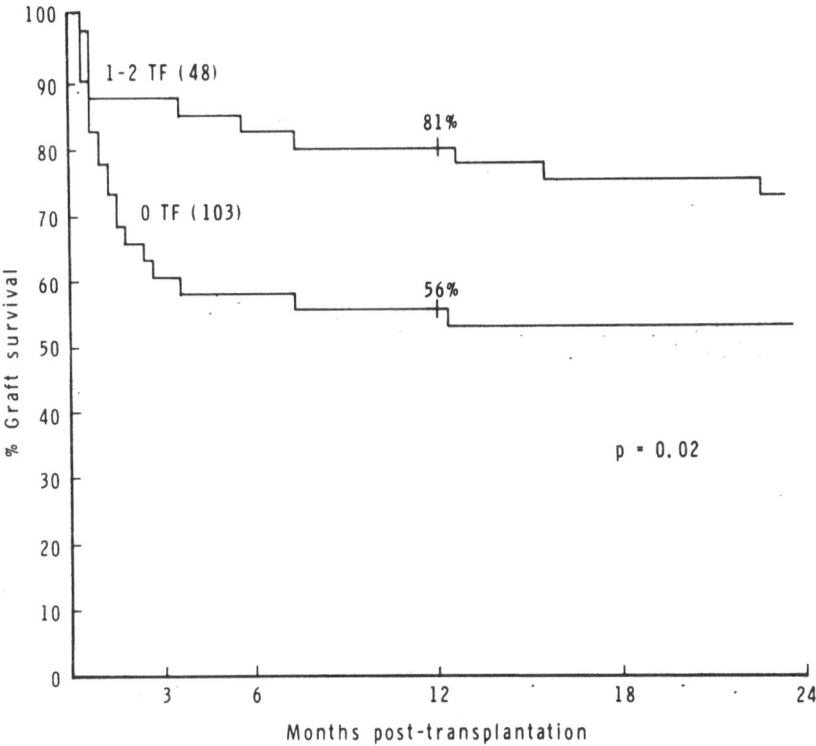

Figure 13.6 The effect of blood transfusion on allograft survival in Oxford. Transfusion of only one or two units of blood pre-transplant produced a significant improvement in graft survival compared to non-transfused patients

expressed that a liberal transfusion policy will lead to an increasing number of patients with high levels of cytotoxic antibodies (Editorial, *Lancet,* 1978). There is also no general agreement on a transfusion protocol which will provide enhancement with a minimal incidence of sensitization. However, recent evidence from primate experiments suggests that platelet transfusions may be effective in producing enhancement without the risks of inducing cytotoxic antibody formation (Borleffs *et al.,* 1982).

Despite the potency of blood transfusion in improving transplant survival the mechanism of action is still unclear. It has been proposed that suppressor cells (van Rood *et al.,* 1978) may be involved or that blood transfusion causes a transient impairment of macrophage activity (Keown and Descamps, 1979). Further research may enable those factors within the blood which are responsible for the transfusion effect to be clearly identified. This would allow the potential complications of elective transfusions with whole blood to be avoided.

13.6 IMMUNOSUPPRESSION

One of the major disappointments in transplantation has been the failure to develop new and more specific immunosuppressive agents over the past 15 years. The majority of transplant patients are still receiving the cocktail of azathioprine and prednisolone developed during the 1960s. In its immuno-logical impact this is blunderbuss therapy and the side-effects, particularly those due to steroids, have been a source of significant morbidity and mortality in transplanted patients. Hypertension, diabetes mellitus, skin changes and avascular necrosis of bone have been common problems, although partially alleviated by the 'low-dose' steroid regime popularized by McGeown (McGeown *et al.,* 1977).

13.6.1 Cyclosporin A

Hundreds of compounds have been tested for immunosuppressive activity *in vitro*, but few have been found to prolong graft survival in experimental animals (Salaman, 1981). The most potent new pharmacological immuno-suppressive agent is cyclosporin A (CS-A). This drug is a metabolite of the soil fungi, *Trichoderma polysporum* and *Cylindrocarpon lucidum*. Initial studies demonstrating the immunosuppressive potential of CS-A *in vitro* (Borel *et al.,* 1976) were followed by experiments in Cambridge confirming that the drug was effective in preventing rejection of organ allografts in animals (Kostakis *et al.,* 1977). The drug was used in initial clinical studies by Professor Calne, reported in the *Lancet,* in 1978 and 1979 (Calne *et al.,* 1978 and 1979; see also Chapter 10). CS-A proved an extremely potent immunosuppressive agent although there were problems with infection when CS-A was combined with other immunosuppressive drugs. In addition CS-A was found to cause both hepatotoxicity and nephrotoxicity. Using a revised protocol of CS-A alone, with bolus i.v. prednisolone to treat rejection, a subsequent report on 32 patients in the Cambridge series showed a one year graft survival of 86% with 11 patients who had not required any steroid treatment (Calne *et al.,* 1981). As CS-A appears to be most effective during the induction phase of the immune response it seems logical to use the drug around the time of transplantation and subsequently to convert patients to conventional immunosuppressive therapy. This approach might achieve maximum immunosuppressive benefit while reducing the risk of side-effects from CS-A. Following the demonstration in canine renal allografts that conversion from CS-A to azathioprine and pred-nisolone could be successfully achieved (Homan *et al.,* 1981) a clinical trial on this basis is now being conducted in Oxford. Patients treated with CS-A for three months, and then converted to azathioprine and prednisolone, are being compared to a control group on azathioprine and prednisolone therapy from the time of transplantation. The preliminary results of this trial show that the group treated with CS-A had graft survival rates at least as good as the conventionally treated patients and it appears likely that a significant benefit from the initial treatment with CS-A will emerge on long-term follow-up.

13.6.2 Monoclonal antisera

The other exciting new development with possibilities for clinical immuno-suppression is the commercial production of monoclonal antibodies and the potential use of these agents in transplant research. This subject was reviewed by Williams in 1979. Monoclonal antibodies are produced by isolating single antibody secreting cells in tissue culture and then fusing them to mouse myeloma cell lines. The resulting hybrid cells grow and divide in culture with the production of large amounts of the specific antibody. Monoclonals against T lymphocyte sub-sets are now available with antibodies to both helper/inducer T cells and suppressor/cytotoxic T cells. These agents offer the prospect of highly specific immunosuppressive therapy and it is hoped that they will soon be available for clinical trial.

13.7 IMMUNOLOGICAL MONITORING

The development of additional forms of immunosuppressive treatment creates the problem of deciding which form of therapy to use in the individual patient. One of the essential developments in transplantation is therefore to devise a form of immunological monitoring, demonstrating whether therapy is effective and, ideally, indicating which agent to use in a specific rejection crisis. Monitoring of lymphocyte and antibody activity in the peripheral blood, although providing valuable information on the mechanism of rejection, has so far failed to gain acceptance in the routine management of transplant patients. The introduction of fine needle aspiration cytology by Häyry and von Willebrand (1978) provides the opportunity of observing cellular infiltration of the graft itself. This is a simple technique in which a 25-gauge spinal needle is introduced into the graft and an aspirate obtained by using constant suction. This process can be repeated, if necessary on a daily basis, without damage to the graft. The cytological preparations are conventionally stained with May-Gruenwald-Giemsa, but we have found that more valuable information can be obtained using monoclonal antibodies to lymphocyte sub-sets and a peroxidase staining technique (Wood *et al.*, 1982). Using fine needle aspiration cytology it may be possible to identify different patterns of rejection with the possibility of tailoring the immunosuppressive regime to the patient's individual requirements.

13.8 CONCLUSIONS

The major breakthrough in transplantation was the establishment of clinical organ grafting at a time when transplant immunology was a developing subject and immunosuppression rudimentary. To a large extent the past 15 years have been a process of catching up and filling in the gaps of our knowledge. It is well recognized that in the treatment of any disease process more is likely to be achieved by a proper application of facts already known than by any specific new development. Transplantation is no exception and if the factors responsible for the 'centre effect' could be identified the overall results of transplantation could be improved considerably. It seems unlikely that developments in tissue matching will have a profound effect on transplantation although a greater knowledge of the significance of cytotoxic antibodies will enable the achievement of a more rational policy for highly sensitised patients. However, it is undoubtedly in the field of immunosuppression, whether by the development of new pharmacological agents or, more likely, by using specific biological reagents, that a real improvement in the results of transplantation can be achieved – a development which will also allow a wider application of transplantation to other disease processes apart from renal failure.

References

Bodmer, W. F., Batchelor, J. R., Bodmer, J. G., Festenstein, H. and Morris, P. J. (eds.) (1978). *Histocompatibility Testing, 1977* (Report of the Seventh International Histocompatibility Workshop and Conference, Oxford). (Copenhagen: Munksgaard)

Borel, J. F., Feurer, C., Gubler, H. U. and Stähelin, H. (1976). Biological effects of cyclosporin A: a new antilymphocytic agent. *Agents Actions*, **6**, 468

Borleffs, J. C. C., Neuhaus, P., van Rood, J. J. and Balner, H., (1982). Platelet transfusions improve kidney allograft survival in rhesus monkeys without inducing cytotoxic antibodies. *Lancet*, **1**, 1117

Calne, R. Y., White, D. J. G., Thiru, S., Evans, D. B., McMaster, P., Dunn, D. C., Craddock, G. N., Pentlow, B. D. and Rolles, K. (1978). Cyclosporin A in patients receiving renal allografts from cadaver donors. *Lancet*, **2**, 1323

Calne, R. Y., Rolles, K., White, D. J. G., Thiru, S., Evans, D. B., McMaster, P., Dunn, D. C., Craddock, G. N., Henderson, R. G., Aziz, S. and Lewis, P. (1979). Cyclosporin A initially as the only immunosuppressant in 34 recipients of cadaveric organs: 32 kidneys, two pancreases and two livers. *Lancet*, **2**, 1033

Calne, R. Y., Rolles, K., White, D. J. G., Thiru, S., Evans, D. B., Henderson, R., Hamilton, D. L., Boone, N., McMaster, P., Gibby, O. and Williams, R. (1981). Cyclosporin A in clinical organ grafting. *Transplant. Proc.*, **13**, 349

Dewar, P. J., Wilkinson, R., Elliott, R. W., Ward, M. K., Kerr, D. N. S., Kenward, D. H., Proud, G and Taylor, R. M. R. (1982). Superiority of B locus matching over other HLA matching in renal graft survival. *Br. Med. J.*, **284**, 779

Editorial (1978). Blood transfusions and renal transplantation. *Lancet*, **2**, 193

van Es, A. A. and Balner, H. (1979). Effect of pre-transplant transfusions on kidney allograft survival. *Transplant. Proc.*, **11**, 127

Festenstein, H., Sachs, J. A., Butterfield, K., Yeatman, N. and Holmes, J. (1981). Collaborative scheme for tissue typing and matching in renal transplantation. XI. Role of HLA-A, B, DR and D matching and other factors on 899 cadaver kidney grafts. *Transplant. Proc.,* **13**, 934

Häyry, P. and von Willebrand, E. (1978). Fine-needle aspiration cytology in the prediction and diagnosis of acute rejection episodes in man. *Proc. Eur. Dial. Transplant Assoc.,* **15**, 335

Homan, W. P., French, M. E., Millard, P. R. and Morris, P. J. (1981). A study of eleven drug regimens using cyclosporin A to suppress renal allograft rejection in the dog. *Transplant. Proc.,* **13**, 397

Jacobs, C., Broyer, M., Brunner, F. P., Brynger, H., Donckerwolcke, R. A., Kramer, P., Selwood, N. H., Wing, A. J. and Blake, P. H. (1981). Combined report on regular dialysis and transplantation in Europe, XI, 1980. *Proc. Eur. Dial. Transplant Assoc.,* **18**, 4

Keown, P. A. and Descamps, B. (1979). Improved renal allograft survival after blood transfusion: a non-specific erythrocyte-mediated immuno-regulatory process? *Lancet,* **1**, 20

Kostakis, A. J., White, D. J. G. and Calne, R. Y. (1977). Prolongation of rat heart allograft survival by cyclosporin A. *IRCS Med. Sci. Library Compendium,* **5**, 280

McGeown, M. G., Kennedy, J. A., Loughridge, W. G. G., Douglas, J., Alexander, J. A., Clarke, S. D., McEvoy, J. and Hewitt, J. C. (1977). One hundred transplants in the Belfast City Hospital. *Lancet,* **2**, 648

Morris, P. J. and Ting, A. (1981). The cross-match in renal transplantation. *Tissue Antigens,* **17**, 75

Opelz, G., Sengar, D. P. S., Mickey, M. R. and Terasaki, P. I. (1973). Effect of blood transfusions on subsequent kidney transplants. *Transplants. Proc.,* **5**, 253

Opelz, G. and Terasaki, P. I. (1980). Dominant effect of transfusions on kidney graft survival. *Transplantation,* **29**, 153

Opelz, G. and Terasaki, P. I. (1982). International study of histocompatibility in renal transplantation. *Transplantation,* **33**, 87

Payne, R., Tripp, M., Weigle, J., Bodmer, W. F. and Bodmer, J. G. (1964). New leukocyte iso-antigen system in man. *Cold Spring Harbor Symp. Quant. Biol.,* **29**, 285

van Rood, J. J., Balner, H. and Morris, P. J., (1978). Blood transfusion and transplantation. *Transplantation,* **26**, 275

Salaman, J. R. (1981). Pharmalogical immunosuppressive agents. In Salaman, J. R. (ed.). *Immunosuppressive Therapy.* pp. 3–18. (Lancaster: MTP Press)

Snell, G. D. (1948). Methods for the study of histocompatibility genes. *J. Genet.,* **49**, 87

Ting, A. and Morris, P. J. (1977). Renal transplantation and B-cell cross-matches with autoantibodies and alloantibodies. *Lancet,* **2**, 1095

Ting, A and Morris, P. J. (1978). Reactivity of autolymphocytotoxic antibodies from dialysis patients with lymphocytes from chronic lymphocytic leukemia (CLL) patients. *Transplantation,* **25**, 31

UK Transplant: Annual Report (1978–1979). UK Transplant Service, Southmead Road, Bristol, UK

Williams, A. F. (1979). Monoclonal antibodies in transplantation research. *Transplantation,* **27**, 152

Wood, R. F. M., Bolton, E. M., Thompson, J. F. and Morris, P. J. (1982). Monoclonal antibodies and fine needle aspiration cytology in detecting renal allograft rejection. *Lancet,* **2**, 278

14

The application of computers to haemodialysis
P. B. Pynsent

14.1 INTRODUCTION

For some time computer systems have been applied specifically to haemo-dialysis centres both for storage and retrieval of patient data and also to clinical problems specific to renal disease (Pollak *et al.*, 1977; Gordon *et al.*, 1979; Masselot *et al.*, 1979; Slama *et al.*, 1979; Bourne *et al.*, 1980; Rorive *et al.*, 1980; Charlton, 1981). A computer system at the Norwich renal unit has been developed that differs from the latter systems in that it provides not only patient data storage and retrieval facilities but also programs designed to control kidney machines during haemodialysis of patients.

The software allows multi-user access to the system. System security is maintained by each user having a password to gain access to data and programs. It is arranged so that all users do not have the same access to data. Thus, for example, the technicians are not able to look at any of the patient data files. Security of data is maintained by changed data files being 'dumped' to tape automatically twice a day.

The computer hardware consists of a Digital PDP11/23 processor with 128k words of memory and two RL01 disc drives. The magnetic tape unit is a Digidata 1740. Information is input and displayed using VT125 visual display units (VDU) modified with touch-sensitive screens (Interaction Systems Inc., Massachusetts USA).

14.2 THE PATIENT DATA SYSTEM

14.2.1 Program selection

All programs are selected from a list of alternatives or 'menus' displayed on the screen of the VDU. Figure 14.1 shows the main menu which is displayed

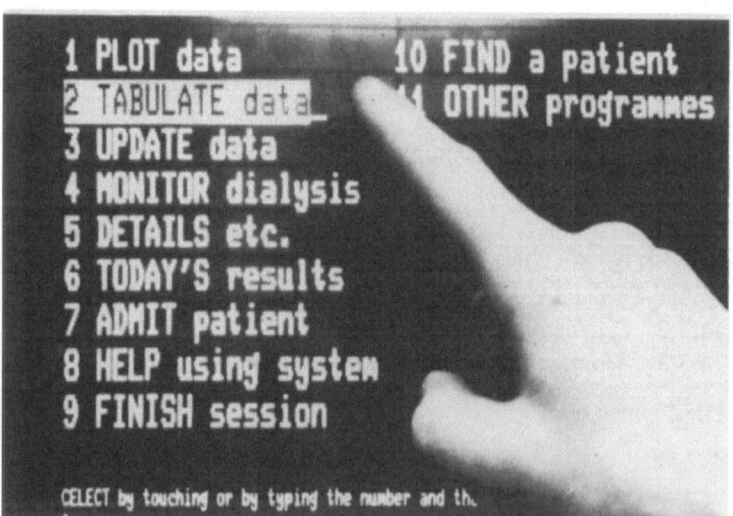

Figure 14.1 The 'main' menu displayed on the screen of the VDU. This menu is displayed upon logging in to the computer and leads to all available functions. Touching an area of the screen selects a function. A 'C' in the bottom left corner appears temporarily as a result of the 'touch'

when a user has gained access to the system by typing in his name and password. This menu is used to select the program function required. When a selected function is completed the system normally returns to this main menu but it is possible to move freely between many of the program functions as will be described later. A program function is selected by touching the display screen or alternatively by typing the number associated with a particular function at the keyboard. In both cases the selection is confirmed by the appropriate section of the screen being displayed in inverse video (Figure 14.1).

14.2.2 Find

Most programs are used for obtaining information about a particular patient; to find a patient the function 'find' is selected from the main menu. The program asks for a clue to the patient being sought (Figure 14.2); either the full six digit hospital number must be touched or typed in or a string of one or more characters. An attempt is then made to match this input with the known patients. Thus if 'J' or 'j' is typed all patients whose names begin with 'J' are sequentially displayed on the screen, each time the user being asked if this is the correct patient until either the reply is 'y' or all matches are exhausted. Although the program 'find' may be selected from the main menu it is usually used from within another function as will be illustrated later. Once a patient is selected, their hospital number, name, date of birth

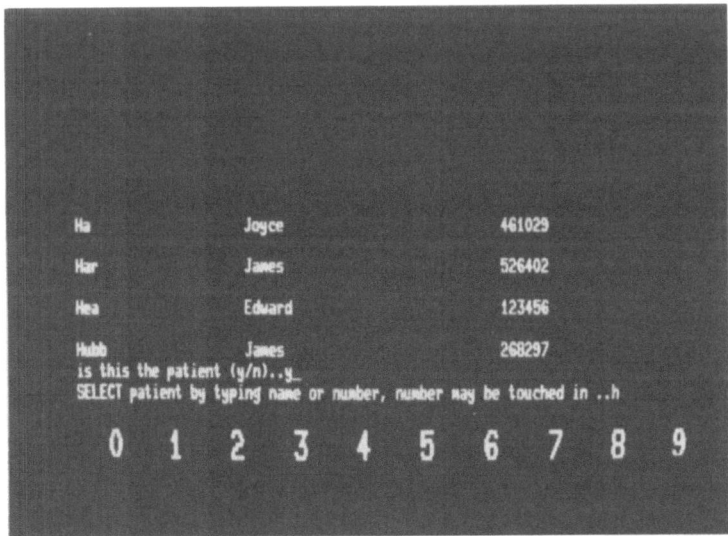

Figure 14.2 The program 'find'. The letter 'h' has been given as the clue to the required patient

and an allergy warning (if appropriate) are displayed at the top of the screen. This patient identity is retained between functions and is only lost when returning to the main menu or when data relevant to the next patient is explicitly requested from the menu.

14.2.3 Admit

When a new patient is admitted to the renal unit they are entered into the computer system by selecting the program 'admit' (Figure 14.3). This program requests the more general details of the patient, such as the date of birth, religion, next of kin etc., and also sets up all the relevant files for the patient on the disc file system. As the hospital number is a unique feature of a patient it must be typed in twice, the first display of the number being deleted before it is requested a second time. If the patient number is already

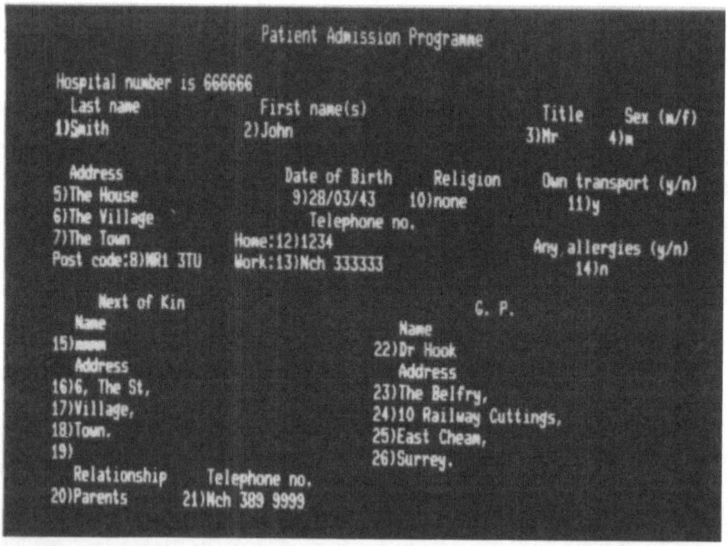

Figure 14.3 The patient admission program

known by the computer it is assumed that the existing patient details are to be edited. Editing of the data is accomplished by moving the screen cursor to the line to be changed using the up/down left/right arrows on the VDU keyboard and then typing in the new information. These personal details may be quickly displayed at any time by selecting 'details' from the main menu (Figure 14.4).

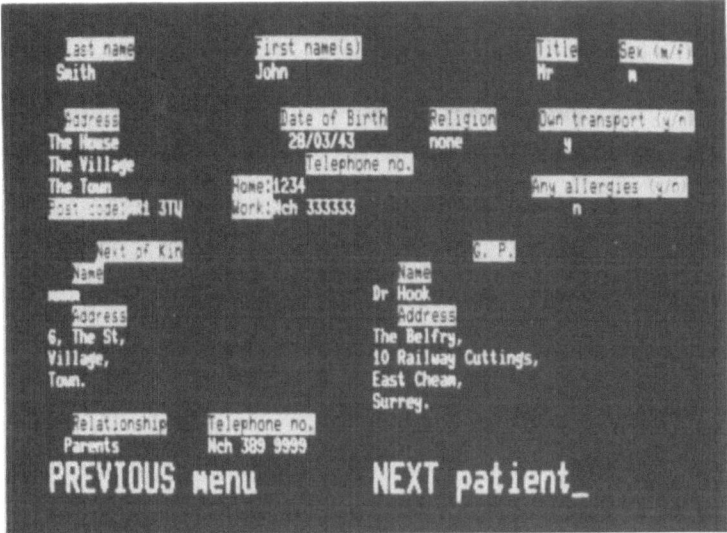

Figure 14.4 A display of a patient's details

14.2.4 Update

The function 'update' is used to enter or edit patient data. After 'update' has been selected from the main menu a patient name is requested (using 'find') and the menu is displayed to select the type of data to be entered (Figure 14.5a). Once the selection is made, a date and time are requested and both are checked, at entry time, for being reasonable values. If an entry already exists for an entered date and time it is assumed that the entry is to be edited. The edit includes the ability to delete complete entries. As far as possible the layout of the selected data type corresponds to the arrangement on the written form (Figure 14.5b). Once again entry and editing of data is accomplished by positioning the cursor with the VDU direction keys. The data collected by 'update' may be looked at in either tabular or plotted form.

14.2.5 Tabulate

'Tabulate' is used to display patient data in a tabular form. Firstly a menu is displayed to select the type of data to be presented (Figure 14.6a) and then, upon selection, the screen is filled with as many forms as possible for that particular data type. For example, for blood biochemistry only four forms can be displayed, whereas for blood pressure and weight there is space for eighteen entries to be displayed simultaneously. At the bottom of the screen three touch pads are annotated, UP, DOWN and FINISH (Figure 14.6b); if

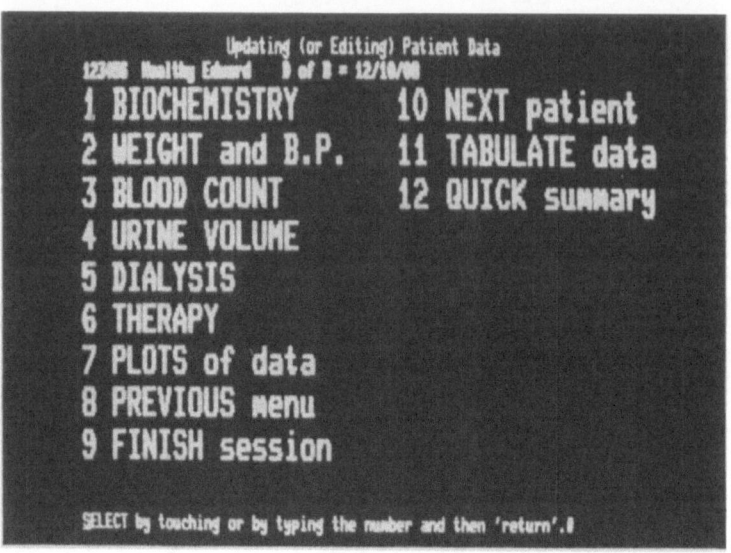

Figure 14.5a   Data-type selection from the update menu

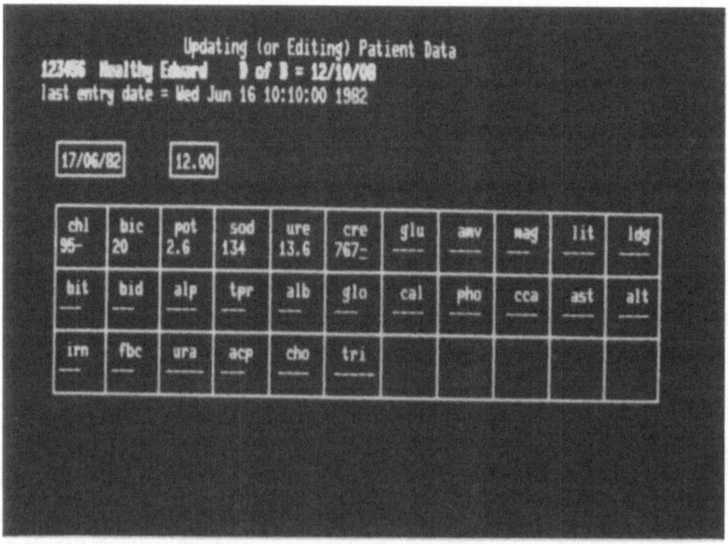

Figure 14.5b   Updating blood biochemistry data

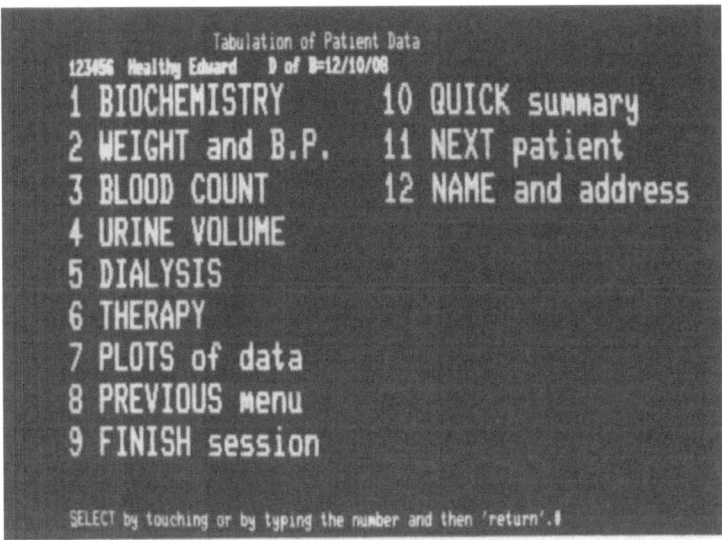

Figure 14.6a The tabulate data menu

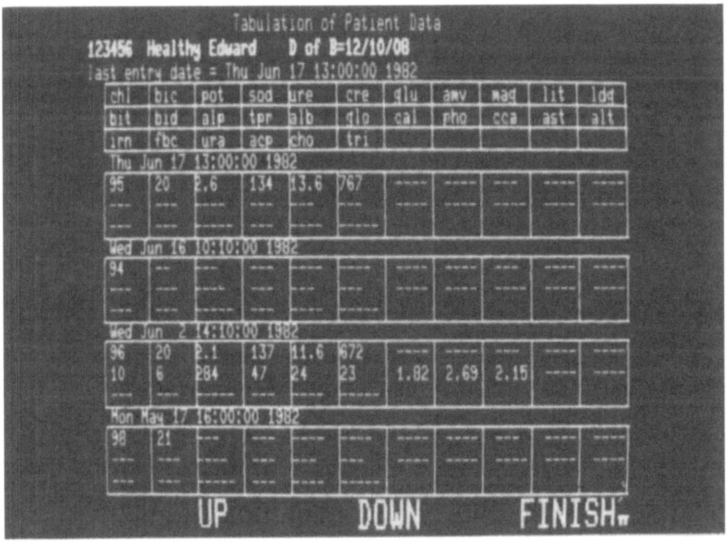

Figure 14.6b Display of patient biochemistry data in tabular form

the finger is held up on the UP the data is scrolled up the screen, older entries being added at the bottom. This scrolling continues until either the finger is removed or all the data has been displayed. In a similar way data can be scrolled forward in time by touching the DOWN pad. When the FINISH is touched then the select data type menu is returned to the screen. Only the centre part of the screen is scrolled, the part at the top displaying the patient identity, and form heading, and the UP/DOWN touch pads at the bottom of the screen are static.

14.2.6 Plot

The patient data can also, and often more usefully, be displayed graphically using the 'plot' function. First, the most commonly required data can be directly plotted by selecting from the menu (Figure 14.7). Secondly, by selection of 'overlay' from the menu up to four different data types may be selected (Figure 14.8a) and superimposed into a single plot (Figure 14.8b). At the bottom of the screen five touch pads are displayed: LEFT, RIGHT, EXPAND, CONTRACT, and END, giving the ability to alter the displayed time window or return to the plot selection menu.

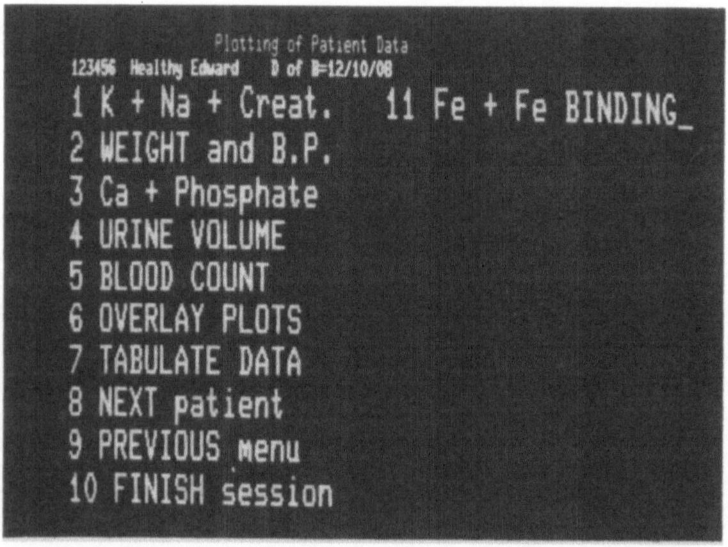

Figure 14.7 The selection menu for the plot function

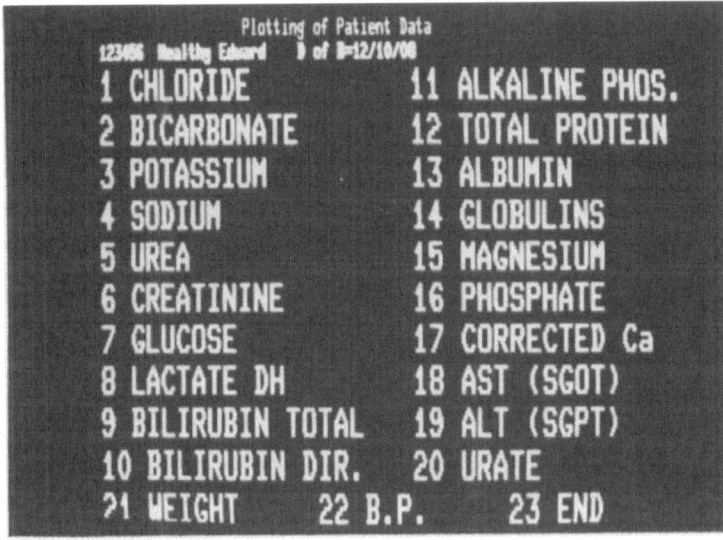

Figure 14.8a   Selection of data to be plotted superimposed

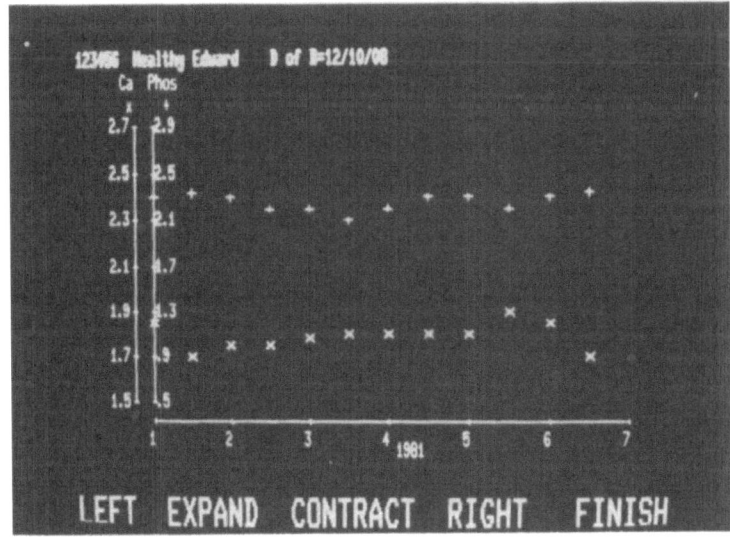

Figure 14.8b   A plot of superimposed data

14.2.7 Other programs

The selection of 'help' from the main menu results in the display of a menu to select help on how to use the various functions. 'Today' gives a summary of all data entered in the last 24 hours for all renal patients. 'Other' programs available are, listing patients names and addresses, mailing facilities, word processing and, for the dieticians, access to the complete McCance and Widdowson's food composition tables (Paul and Southgate, 1978) as extended by the Dunn Nutrition Unit at Cambridge (Wiles *et al.*, 1980).

14.3 COMPUTER CONTROLLED DIALYSIS

14.3.1 The hardware for dialysis control

The prime requirement for computer-controlled dialysis is a suitable dialysis machine. The Seratron (Cordis-Dow International Ltd., Slough, UK) is believed to be the only dialysis machine available at present that provides a suitable interface to a computer. This machine (Figure 14.9) allows control over the ultrafiltration rate and dialysate concentration together with setting of various alarm levels. It additionally allows interrogation of the machine for the current status, switch settings and alarm conditions. The manufacturers also supply a network controller system to allow many Seratrons to be connected to a single port of the controlling computer. All terminals and network controllers connect to the main computer using

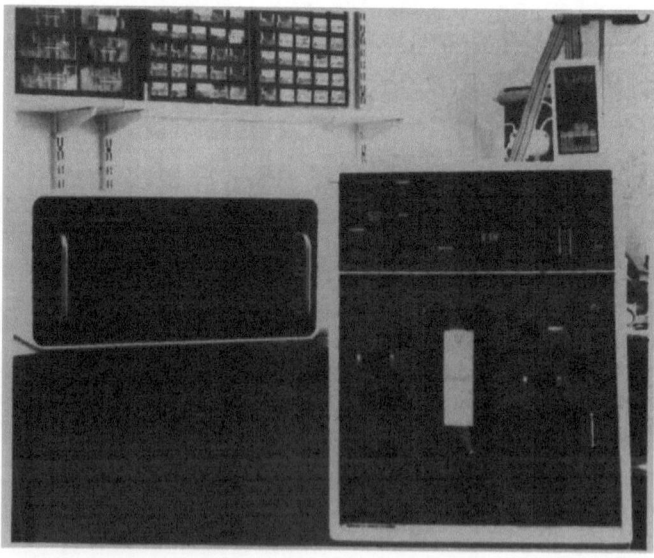

Figure 14.9 The Seratron dialysis machine with its hand-held remote programmer (above) and the network controller (right)

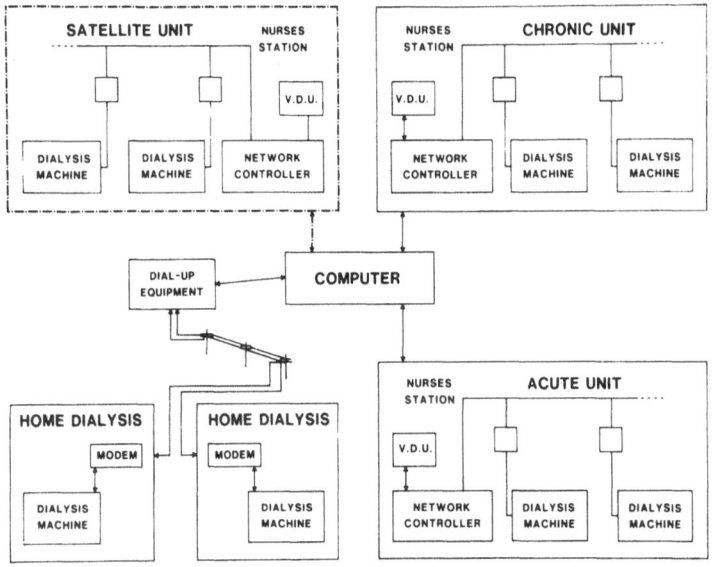

Figure 14.10   The arrangement of the central computer to the various dialysis centres

standard RS-232 ports (Figure 14.10) remote sites are connected via Post Office lines through multiplexer and modem units (Racal-Milgo, Hants., UK).

It is important to ensure that the patient identified by the nurse on the VDU is connected to the correct dialysis machine. This is accomplished by the nurse having to confirm the patient identity at the bedside using the remote programmer (Figure 14.10).

14.3.2   Setting dialysis parameters

Data for describing and controlling dialysis is entered by selecting the 'dialysis' option of the 'update' menu. This option displays the currently prescribed dialysis parameters in the upper part of the screen below the patient identification (Figure 14.11); changes to the data are made at the bottom of the screen. The central part of the display is used to display the time course of the current dialysis model. Four model options are supported at the moment; 0 – no model. 1 – linear model, 2 – exponential decay and 3 – sequential dialysis. Initially the new data (lower part of the screen) is set to the existing values. Using the direction keys of the VDU the dialysis data can be edited. If the model or the model parameters are changed then the central graphics area of the screen is correspondingly altered.

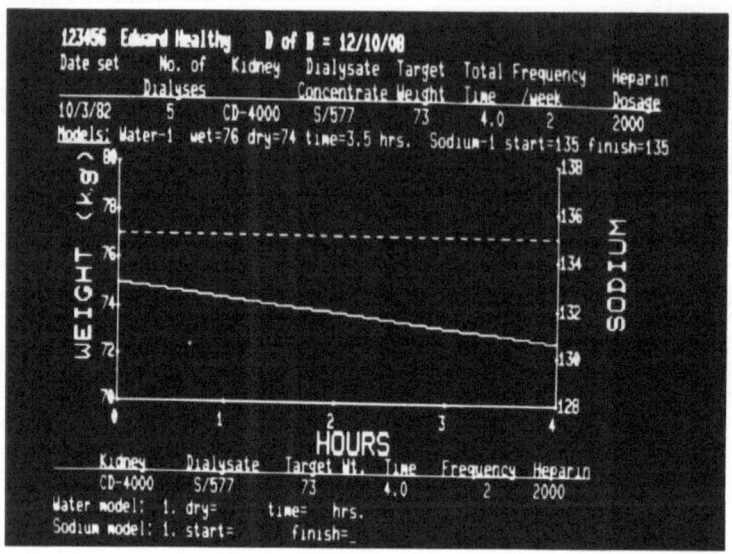

Figure 14.11 Updating the dialysis prescription

14.3.3 Monitoring and control of dialysis

Selection of the 'monitor' function from the main menu allows the progress of dialysis to be monitored and may also be used to initiate computer control of dialysis. Firstly the site to be monitored is requested (Figure 14.12). This allows any terminal to monitor dialysis at any site on the computer system although only one terminal may control dialysis at a specific site. The software knows which terminal should have control over a given site but because it is possible to 'cross wires' a check is always made that the terminal location agrees with the programmed site. Once a site has been selected the current state of the dialysis patients at the selected site is displayed (Figure 14.13). The positions may be in an active (dialysis in progress) state or passive state. Touching a displayed position that is in an active state produces information about the progress of dialysis; for positions that have computer-controlled machines the information may be quite detailed. Touching a position that is in a passive state starts the set up procedure for connecting a patient to a machine. If the patient is to be dialysed with a machine that is computer controllable a second task is initiated to set up and control the machine. This latter program will then communicate with the 'monitor' program. The independence of the dialysis control program means that programs to control new machines with different protocols may easily be installed into the system with a need for only a new controlling program.

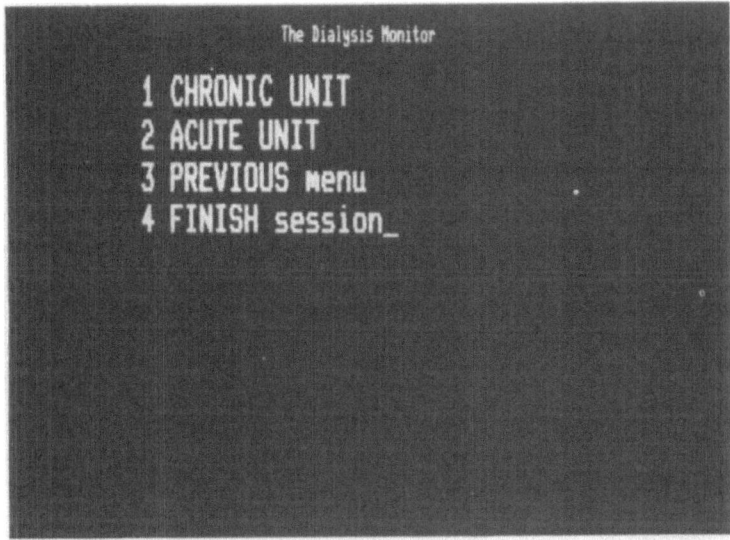

Figure 14.12 Selection of the dialysis centre to be monitored

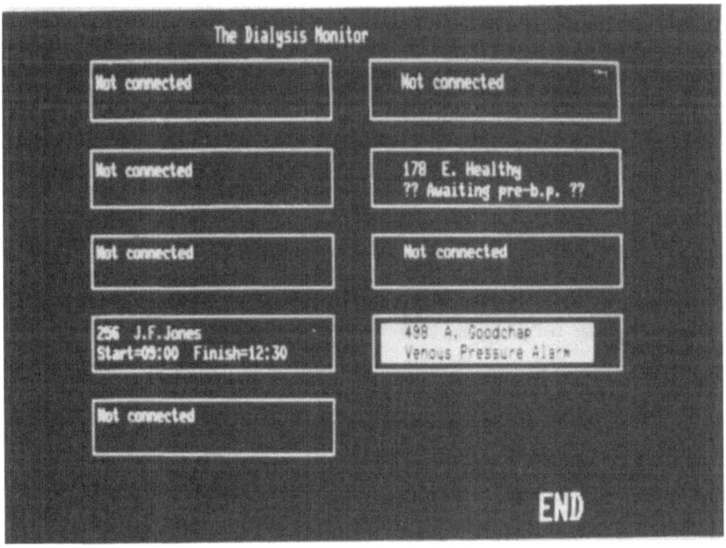

Figure 14.13 Current state of the selected unit. Note that one station has a flashing inverse video display as it is in an alarm condition

14.4 DISCUSSION

The objective at the Norwich renal unit was to produce a computer controlled dialysis system; but at the same time a patient database system has been
developed which is easy to use and helps the physician to make clinical
decisions and nurses to implement these decisions. The computer control of
dialysis is in an early stage but it is believed that the advent of this control
over dialysis will allow the application of sophisticated modelling
procedures leading to improved patient care. Although the software has
been designed for the easy addition of dialysis machines of different manufacture, it is hoped that at this early stage the manufacturers will be encouraged to produce machines with a standard hardware interface and
software protocol. The computer system provides the tools for detailed
monitoring and control of dialysis at remote sites and this implies
economies in terms of reduced staffing at these sites whilst still maintaining
a high standard of patient care.

References

Bourne, J. R., Hamel, B., Giese, D., Woyce, G. M., Lawrence, P. L., Ward, J. W.
    and Teschan, P. E. (1980). The EEG analysis system of the national cooperative
    dialysis study. *IEEE Trans. Biomed. Eng., 27*, 656

Charlton, B. A. (1981). A nurse-managed computerised medical record system in
    dialysis and transplantation. *Proc. Eur. Dial. Transplant Nurses Assoc., 9*, 132

Gordon, M., de Wardener, H. E., Gower, P. E. and Curtis, J. R. (1979). The use of
    computer graphics in a maintenance haemodialysis unit. (*Abstract*) *Eur. Dial.
    Transplant Assoc., 16*, 33

Masselot, J. P., Adhemar, J. P., Laederich, J., Degoulet, P. and Kleinknechkt, D.
    (1979). Utilisation du système informatique DIAPHANE pour la surveillance
    des patients traités par hémodialyse à domicile. *J. Urol. Nephrol. (Paris), 85*,
    963

Paul, A. A. and Southgate, D. A. T. (1978). *McCance and Widdowson's – The
    Composition of Foods.* (London: Her Majesty's Stationery Office; Amsterdam
    and New York: Elsevier/North Holland)

Pollak, V. E., Buncher, R and Donovan, R. (1977). On-line computerised data
    handling system for treating patients with renal disease. *Arch. Intern. Med.,
    137*, 446

Rorive, G., Gyselynck-Mambourg, A. M., Sabatier, J. and Gentinne, J. L. (1980).
    Computer-assisted medical care in a haemodialysis unit. *Med. Inf. (London), 5*,
    227

Slama, G., Klein, J. C., Delage, A., Rottembourg, J., Marouani, A. and Jacobs, C.
    (1979). The use of the artificial pancreas in uremic diabetic patients. *Horm.
    Metab. Res. Suppl., Part 8*, 178

Wiles, S. J., Nettleton, P. A., Black, A. E. and Paul, A. A. (1980). The nutritional
    composition of some cooked dishes eaten in Britain: a supplementary food
    composition table. *J. Hum. Nut., 34*, 189

15

The morphology of the peritoneum with special reference to peritoneal dialysis
J. W. Dobbie,
M. A. Zaki and L. S. Wilson

15.1   INTRODUCTION

Peritoneal morphology has not previously engendered much interest. A few
basic studies of this tissue have been made in rodents, yet despite unlimited
access to normal human peritoneum at routine surgical operations little is
known of the ultrastructure of the peritoneal mesothelium and subjacent
structures in man.

In a previous paper (Dobbie *et al.*, 1981) we have commented on this
surprising lack of knowledge in relation to the increasing use of continuous
ambulatory peritoneal dialysis (CAPD) as a life-maintaining procedure.
Since this form of dialysis is in its infancy, we are as yet unaware of the
longterm effect on the morphology of the peritoneum of continuous
exposure to dialysis solutions of varying tonicity, possibly contaminated
with trace amounts of foreign substances and of the sequelae of repeated
episodes of bacterial or 'chemical' peritonitis.

This paper is an account of our findings obtained by light, transmission
and scanning electron microscopy (TEM and SEM) in a morphological
study of normal peritoneum in rodent and man, and of the peritoneum after
exposure to dialysis solutions.

15.2   MATERIAL AND METHODS

15.2.1   Specimens

Small portions of peritoneum (25–100 mm²) were removed from either the
anterior abdominal wall (parietal) or serosal surface of an organ (visceral)
with the minimum of handling or trauma. Samples of normal human
peritoneum were obtained at routine surgical operations. Samples were also
taken from the parietal peritoneum of uraemic patients during insertion of a
peritoneal catheter and from patients subjected to CAPD during removal or
replacement of the catheter. Specimens of parietal peritoneum were also
taken from normal stock experimental animals (rat and mouse).

15.2.2   En face silver stained preparations

Silver staining of the peritoneal surface was performed using a modification
of the method of Poole *et al.* (1958). Specimens were immersed in an 0.25%
solution of silver nitrate for 1 minute before transfer to a solution
containing 3% cobalt bromide and 1% ammonium bromide for 3 minutes.
After several rinses in 5% glucose the tissue was fixed in 10% buffered
formalin for 2 hours. Very thin shavings of tissue were then cut from the
surface with a razor blade, cleared in dioxane for 2 hours and mounted flat
on glass slides.

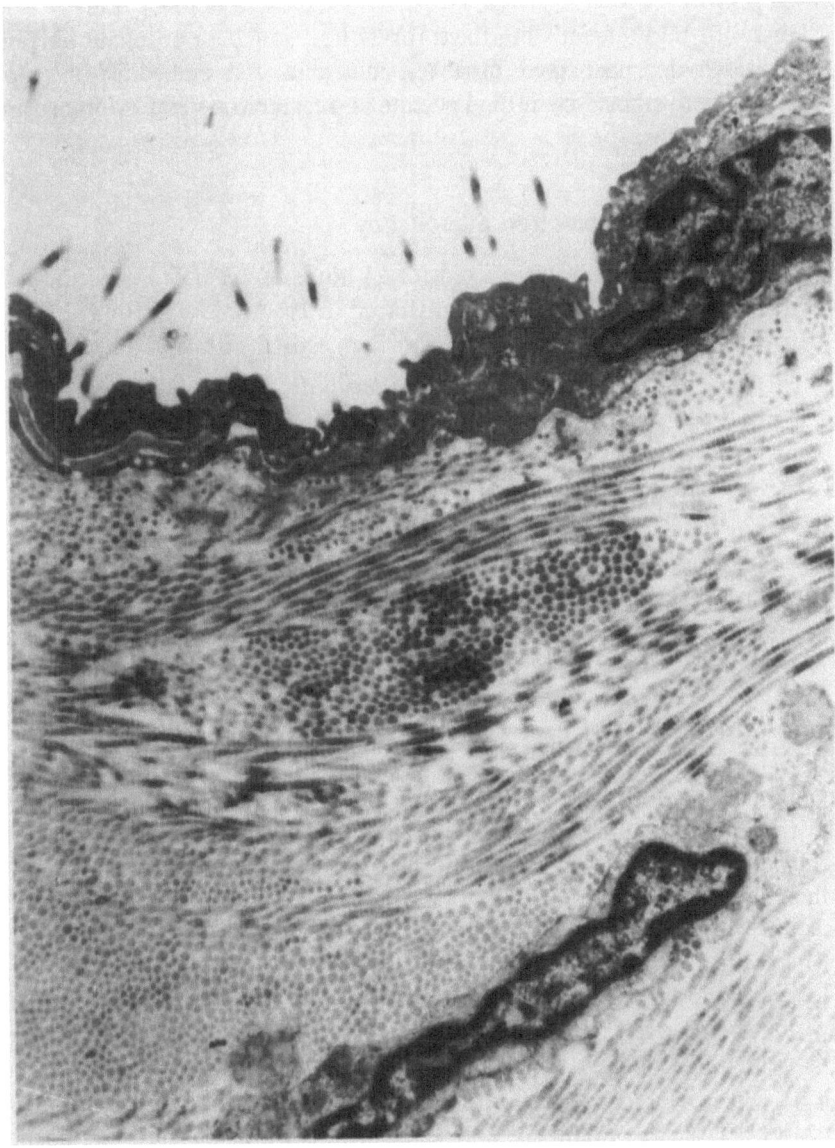

Figure 15.1 Section through normal human peritoneum showing thin mesothelial cells resting on an indistinct basal lamina. Microvilli can be seen arising from the free surface. In the subjacent tissue, interwoven bundles of collagen fibres lie in a loose ground substance. A fibroblast is present near the lower border of the section. Magnification × 12320

15.2.3 Transmission electron microscopy

Samples of peritoneum were fixed for 24 hours in 2% phosphate-buffered glutaraldehyde, post-fixed in 1% osmic acid and embedded in epon. Sections were stained by uranyl acetate and lead citrate and examined in a JEM 6A microscope.

15.2.4 Scanning electron microscopy

Samples of peritoneum were fixed for 24 hours in 2% buffered glutaraldehyde containing 7.5% sucrose, transferred to 1% osmic acid for 1-2 hours, before critical point drying. They were then coated with gold and examined in an ISI III–A scanning electron microscope.

15.3 RESULTS

15.3.1 En face silver stained preparations

In preparations of peritoneum from normal man and rodents, the borders of mesothelial cells were delineated by deposition of the silver stain to show a mosaic pattern of polygonal cells in unbroken contact. Each cell possessed 5-7 relatively straight sides allowing contact with 5-7 adjacent cells.

15.3.2 Transmission electron microscopy

In general the ultrastructural findings in specimens from normal rodent, normal man and uraemic patients were closely similar. Sections vertical to the peritoneal surface showed thin, flat, mesothelial cells resting on a rather indistinct basal lamina (Figure 15.1). The cells were thicker in the central region where the nucleus was situated than at the periphery (Figure 15.2). Microvilli arose from the free mesothelial surface being up to 2.5 μm in length (Figures 15.1 and 15.2). In most sections, cell junctions were sloped with one cell overlapping the other. Junctional complexes were observed between cells (Figure 15.3). Close to the mesothelial surface, membranes of adjoining cells were fused to give the zonula occludens or tight junction. At a deeper level was found the zonula adhaerens while the third and deepest element of the junctional complex was the macula adhaerens or desmosome. Below the desmosome the intercellular clefts showed fusiform dilatations, side branches and interdigitation of cell processes. The mesothelial cell cytoplasm contained numerous mitochondria, elements of rough endoplasmic reticulum, Golgi apparatus and lysosomes (Figure 15.2). The cytoplasm was packed with a great many vesicles of various form and size some of which were coated. Perhaps the most striking feature of the mesothelial cells was the profusion of micropinocytic vesicles which lined both the inner and outer surfaces (Figure 15.2).

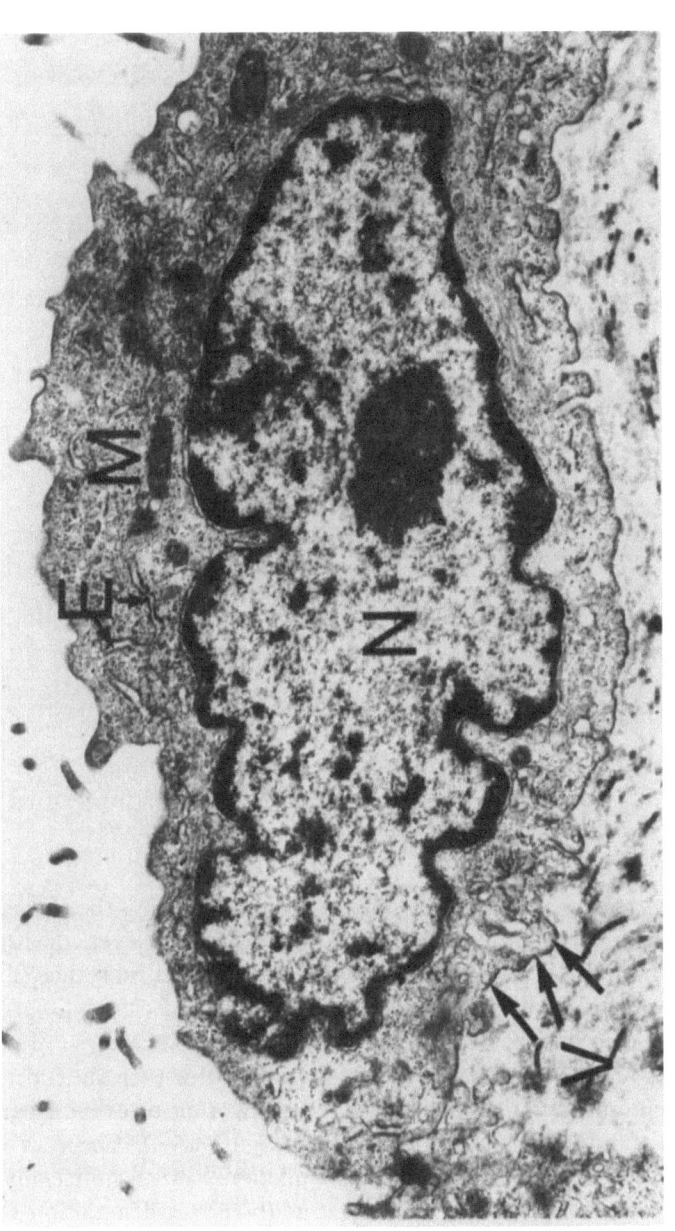

Figure 15.2 Section through normal parietal mesothelium demonstrating the typical elongated convoluted nucleus (N), mitochondria (M), rough endoplasmic reticulum (E) and micropinocytic vesicles (V). Magnification × 16 100

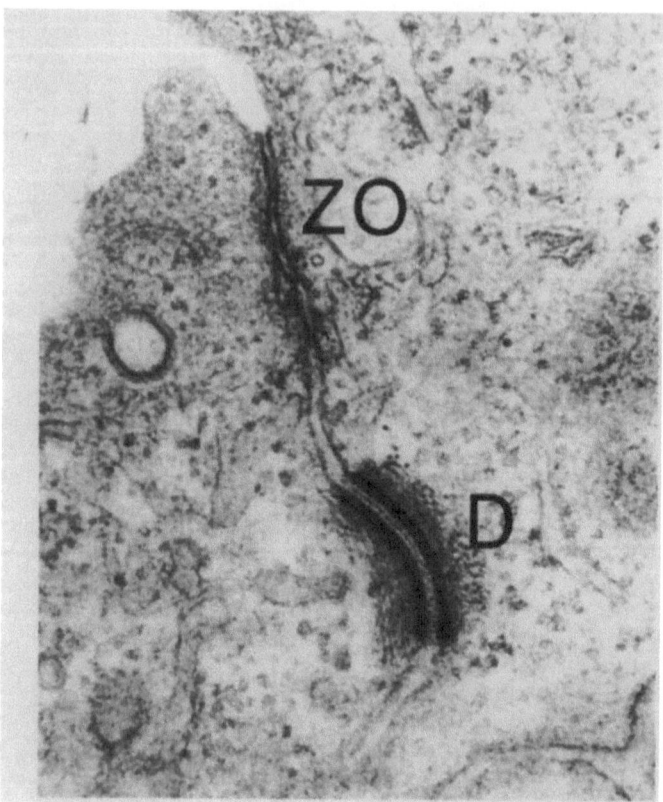

Figure 15.3 Shows elements in an uraemic patient of the junctional complex between two mesothelial cells. The complex nearest the free surface is the zonula occludens (ZO), the innermost complex is a desmosome (D) or macula adhaerens. Magnification × 69 370

In parietal peritoneum and visceral peritoneum covering the alimentary canal, the tissue between the mesothelium and the muscle layer consisted of interwoven bundles of collagen fibres in a loose ground substance (Figure 15.1). In some sites there ran a discontinuous band of elastic tissue. The main cell types in this region were fibroblasts and mast cells.

In animals and patients exposed to dialysis fluid for even short periods, the most striking finding in the mesothelium was that of cellular oedema with dilution and dispersion of organelles (Figure 15.4). The cells often appeared to be more attenuated while microvilli were noticeably less numerous (Figure 15.5). In some specimens there was denudation of the mesothelial cell layer. Alterations observed in the subjacent tissues were those of oedema and increased numbers of fibroblasts and mast cells. In specimens obtained from patients whose catheters were removed because of peritonitis (Figure 15.6) the mesothelial layer was frequently missing, being

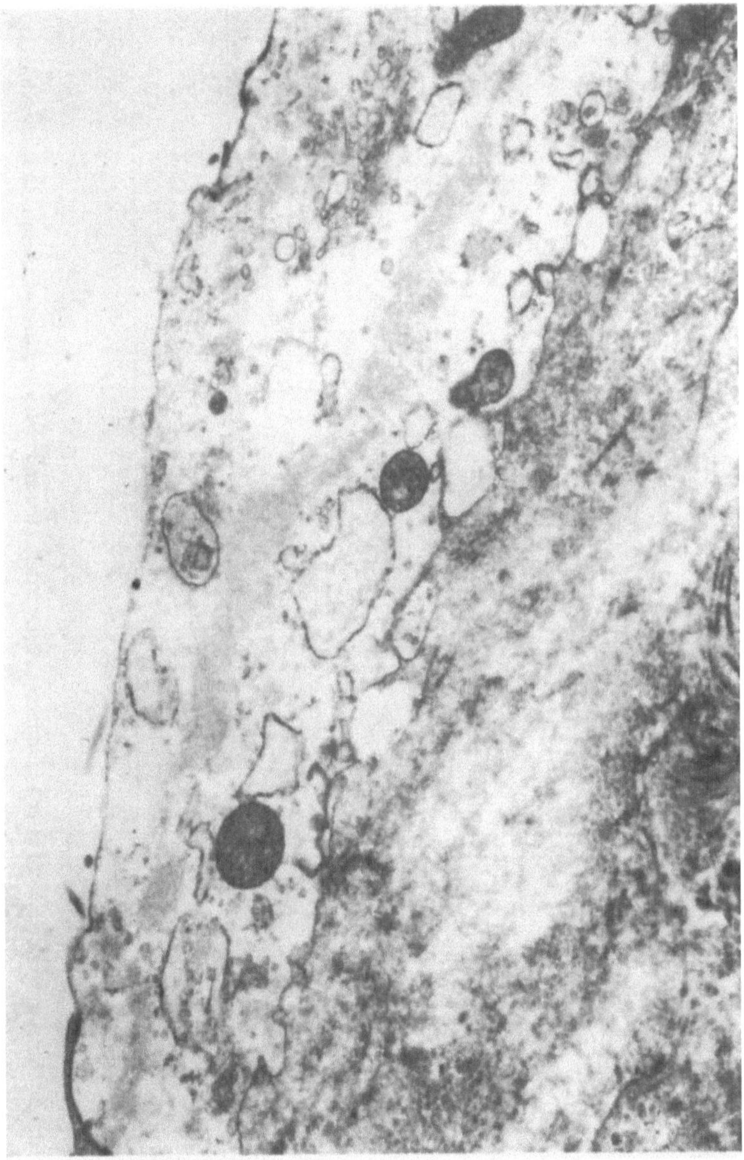

Figure 15.4 Oedematous mesothelium showing dispersion and disorganization of cytoplasmic structures. Parietal peritoneum from patient after 3 months on CAPD. Magnification ×23 625

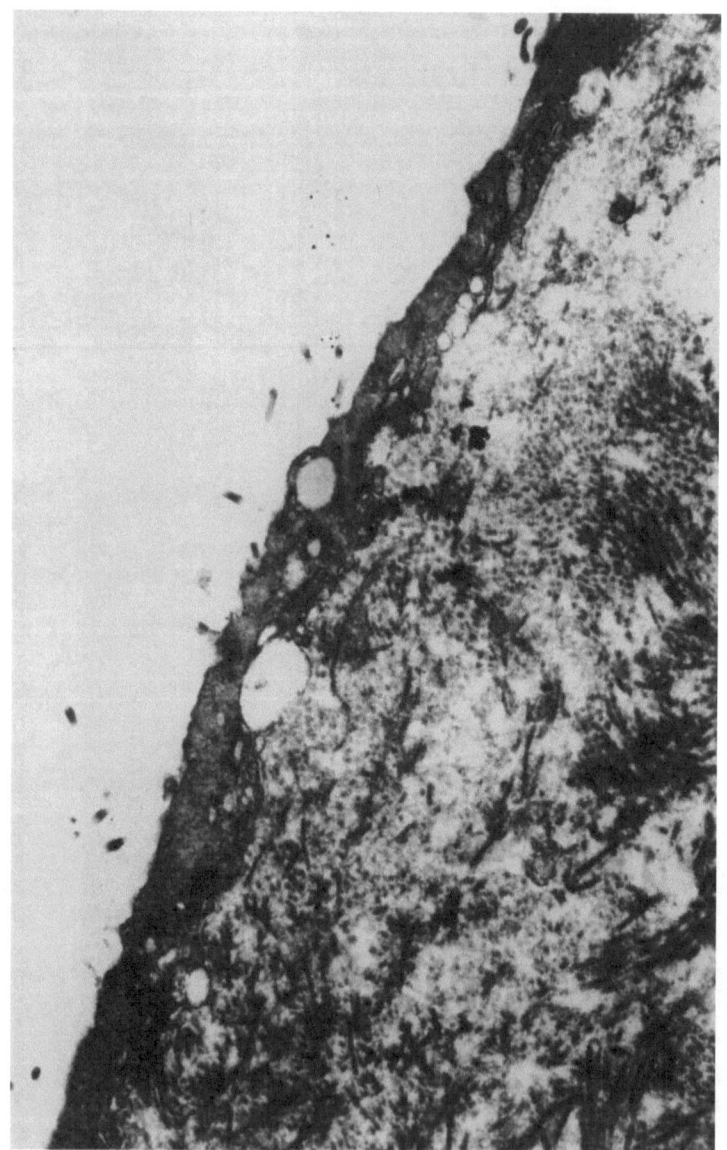

Figure 15.5   Parietal peritoneum from a patient after 1 month on CAPD. Attenuated and rather featureless mesothelium showing few stunted micro-villi. Magnification ×8400

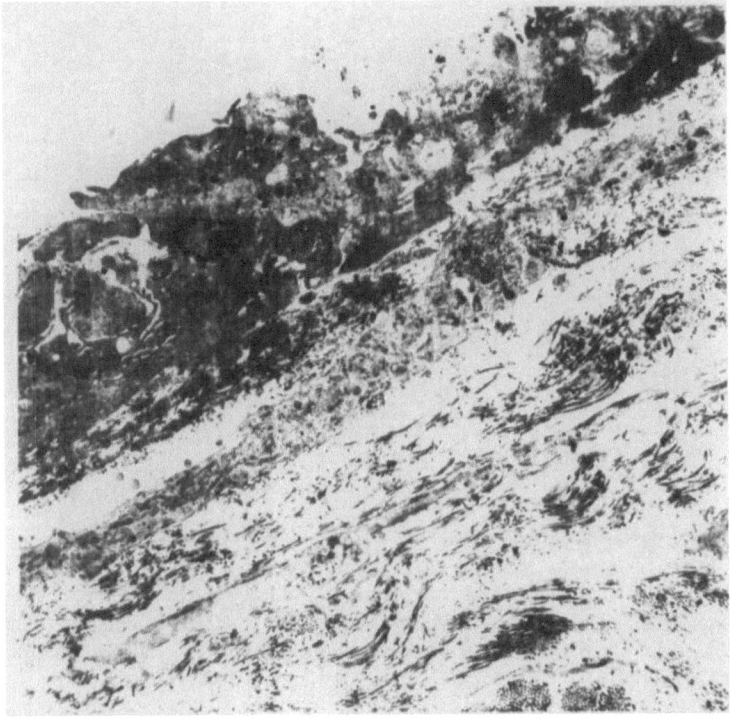

Figure 15.6 Section through parietal peritoneum of patient on CAPD, whose catheter was removed because of repeated episodes of peritonitis. The free surface is lined by degenerate mesothelial and inflammatory cells. A fibroblast lies immediately below in an oedematous stroma. Magnification × 4620

replaced by a layer of amorphous debris, while the underlying tissue was heavily infiltrated with polymorphs, eosinophils and mast cells.

15.3.3 Scanning electron microscopy

This technique demonstrated most effectively the rich profusion of micro-villi which carpeted normal mesothelium (Figure 15.7 and 15.8). Although the cell surfaces lay hidden beneath the microvillous carpet, a perceptible variation in contour and density of microvilli betrayed the polygonal pavemented arrangement of the underlying mesothelial cells. In some areas where the microvilli were less profuse the actual mesothelial cell surface could be seen through appropriate gaps (Figure 15.8). Here were visible small, round holes which represented the opercula or openings of the micro-pinocytic vesicles.

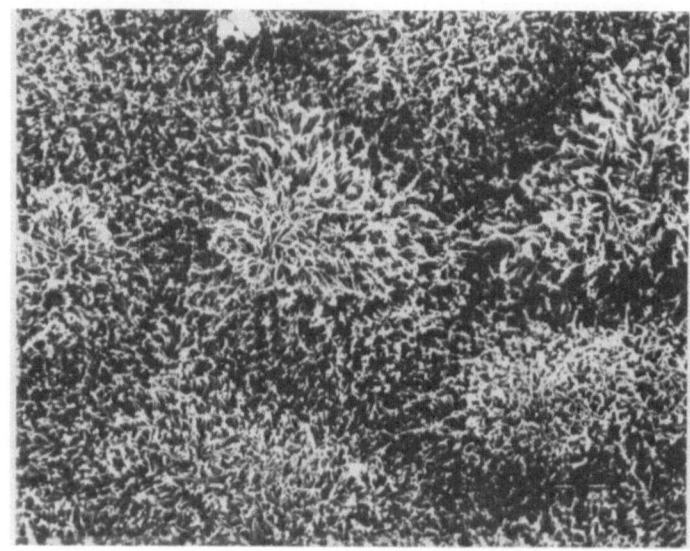

Figure 15.7   SEM of normal rat parietal peritoneum showing the thick carpet of microvilli which obscure the underlying mesothelial cell surfaces. The rounded contours and connecting depressions delineate the individual positions of the mesothelial cells beneath. Magnification × 2250

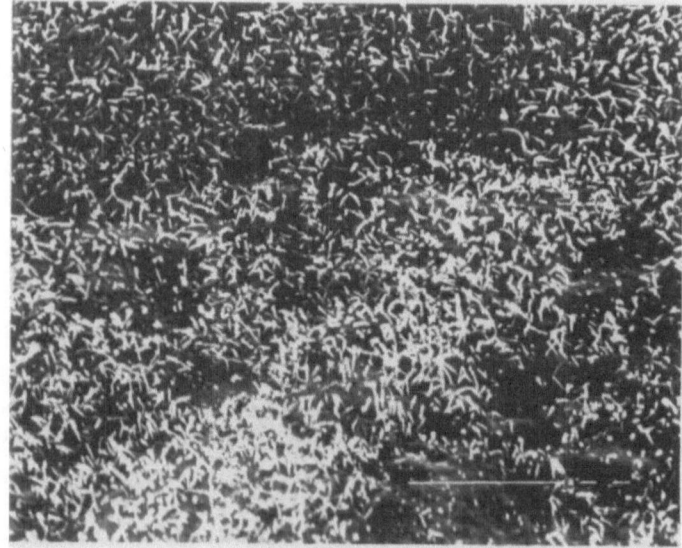

Figure 15.8   SEM of normal human parietal peritoneum. In this biopsy the microvilli are less profuse revealing the surface of the mesothelial cells. Magnification × 1987

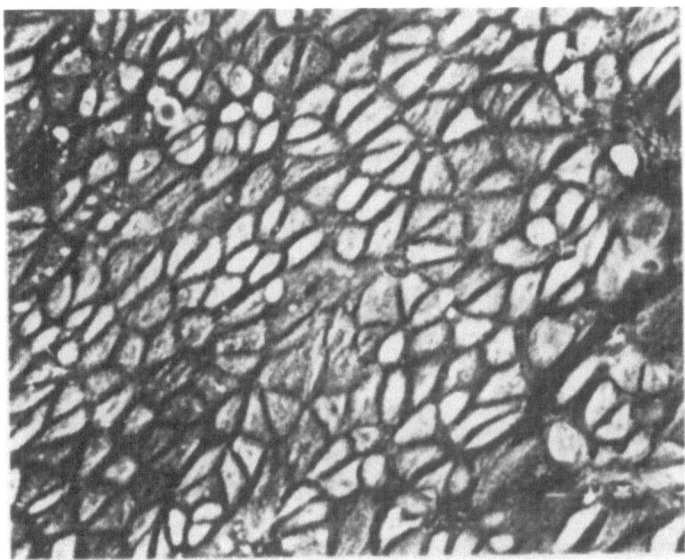

Figure 15.9 SEM of biopsy of parietal peritoneum from patient on CAPD for 20 months. In contrast to Figures 15.7 and 15.8 the microvillous carpet is thin revealing an accentuated, almost dissected, pavementation pattern of polygonal mesothelial cells. Magnification × 262

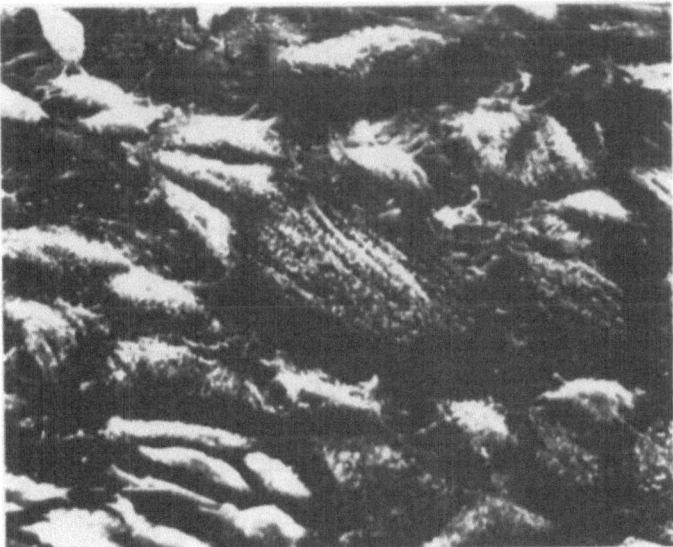

Figure 15.10 A higher magnification of the same specimen as in Figure 15.9 shows the general untidiness of the mesothelial surface where the cells are humped up due to retraction and stretching of the peripheral margins of their cytoplasm. The paucity and stunting of microvilli contrast sharply with the appearances in Figures 15.7 and 15.8. Magnification × 562

In rodents, scanning electron microscopy showed obvious changes in the surface characteristics of the mesothelial cell layer after only 24 hours exposure to hypertonic peritoneal dialysis fluid. The main finding was retraction and decrease in density of the microvilli to reveal the pavemented nature of the underlying mesothelial cells. More prolonged exposure to dialysis fluid was accompanied by further reduction in the 'pile' of the microvillous carpet and exposure of the mesothelium. Similar changes were encountered in biopsies obtained from patients after 1 week to 20 months on CAPD (Figures 15.9 and 15.10). In patients with peritonitis, specimens of peritoneum frequently showed barren, roughened, ribbed or woven-textured surfaces denuded of epithelium (Figure 15.11).

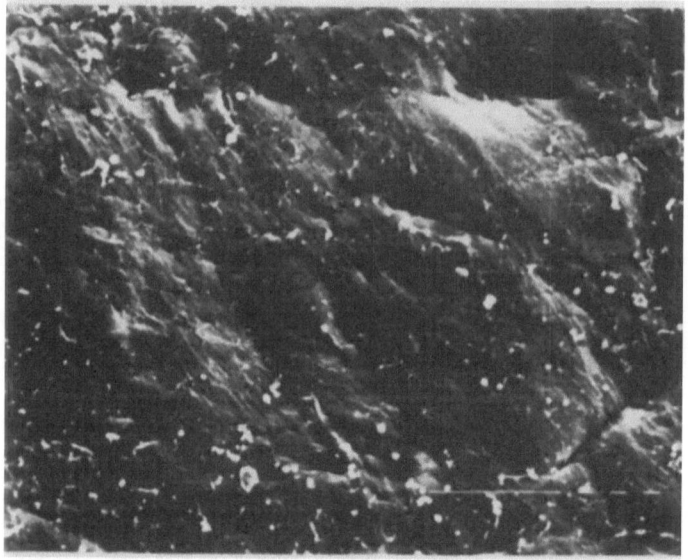

Figure 15.11 SEM of biopsy of parietal peritoneum in a patient whose catheter was removed because of repeated severe episodes of peritonitis. This shows a barren, rather 'glaciated' surface, denuded of its mesothelial cell layer. Magnification × 169

15.4 DISCUSSION

Observations made in these initial investigations indicate that the ultra-structural and surface characteristics of the normal mesothelium are broadly similar in rodents, normal man and uraemic patients. Exposure to dialysis fluid in both experimental animals and in CAPD patients caused significant changes. These consisted largely of cellular oedema, peripheral attenuation of the mesothelial cytoplasm, retraction and loss of microvilli and areas of cellular denudation. However, the information gathered so far must be viewed as random observations. Further detailed examination of larger numbers of specimens of peritoneum from patients with varying periods on CAPD is required before one may attempt to categorize and evaluate the progression of changes which may result from continuous exposure to dialysis fluid.

Scanning electron microscopy demonstrated most effectively the vast increase in surface area conferred on normal mesothelium by its profuse covering of microvilli. Whether they contribute significantly to the passage of fluid and solutes through the mesothelium and whether their apparent diminution or loss with exposure to dialysis fluid has an appreciable effect on the process of dialysis is as yet unknown. Likewise the role of the ubiquitous micropinocytic vesicles in the transport of materials across the mesothelial cell layer demands further study. The integrity of the junctional complexes following CAPD is important with respect to the efficiency of dialysis and as a factor in the process of mesothelial cell denudation on exposure to dialysis fluid.

These ultrastructural studies have shown that one cannot assume that the mesothelium is simply a lining cell devoid of any great functional activity or that it lacks an active role in the passage of material across its cytoplasm. The provision of significant numbers of mitochondria, well developed Golgi apparatus and lysosomes tend to support the impression that the mesothelial cell is not merely the cellular lining of a passive membrane system.

References

Dobbie, J. W., Zaki, M. and Wilson, L. (1981). Ultrastructural studies of the peritoneum with special reference to chronic ambulatory peritoneal dialysis. *Scot. Med. J.,* **26,** 213

Poole, J. C. G., Sanders, A. G. and Florey, H. W. (1958). The regeneration of aortic endothelium. *J. Pathol. Bacteriol.,* **75,** 133

Discussion

A. C. Kennedy: It is true to say that the best culling of kidneys for transplantation occurs nearest the transplant unit. Is there therefore a case for increasing the number of transplant units? Would that be an effective way of improving the numbers done?

R. Y. Calne: Well it might do. I am a little worried about that as a solution because to have an effective unit really needs a minimum of two consultant surgeons doing transplantation. In Cambridge, we have two consultant surgeons and three registrars who do transplants. There is also a general interest in transplantation and the whole of the research in my department is concerned with transplantation. We have nurses experienced in it. We have a transplant co-ordinator.

Satellite transplant centres will dilute this concentration of interest and expertise, and I am a little doubtful whether increasing the number of transplants units all over the country will improve results. It might increase the number of cases being transplanted but I doubt very much that it will improve the results.

We have a Regional centre for neurosurgery, for radiotherapy, why not for transplantation? That has always been the Department of Health's policy, and I think a wise policy.

G. Pincherle (DHSS): It has been suggested that as well as, or perhaps instead of, a Regional transplant coordinator, there might be a transplant coordinator in a District General Hospital, who would not be full-time but part-time and perhaps could be a respected local consultant. What are Professor Calne's views?

Calne: I would welcome it very much. It would be very valuable to have, in a District Hospital, someone who is prepared to spend a bit of time and effort persuading his colleagues that to help a patient whom they cannot actually see is still helping a patient and is fulfilling medical ethics. I think this thought is the main reason why help is not forthcoming; people ask 'where is this patient?'. But in fact the patient is usually in Norwich and the donor is usually in Cambridge!

D. Benoliel (National Federation of Kidney Patients Associations): I asked this question nearly 2 years ago and I want to know if there has been any further work done on ways of changing patients from conventional immunosuppression to cyclosporin A and vice versa?

Calne: Yes. It seems that it is usually not too difficult to move patients from one form of therapy to another. We have moved quite a number of patients, maybe ten, from conventional therapy to cyclosporin A. Of course patients who develop rejection on cyclosporin A are routinely changed to azathioprine and steroids.

The only patients that we have changed have been patients who have been getting complications from azathioprine and steroids because we feel reluctant to rock the boat if somebody is doing outstandingly well on conventional therapy. Azathioprine is a good drug too.

Kennedy: I am not quite clear what are the limiting factors preventing the wider use of cyclosporin A now; why we are still at the stage of having controlled trials when the results seem so extremely good?

Calne: We are not that far away. The Sandoz Company had a preliminary look at the randomized trial but it will not be possible to give a definitive result until another year has gone by. All the patients who have come into the trial now need to be followed up. Sandoz feel already that the results are sufficiently encouraging, as are the results in North America and Australia, to market the drug, possibly towards the end of the year. Manufacture of the drug requires a considerable tooling up process on fermentation, and particularly on purification. I do not know how expensive the drug is likely to be. I have been trying to persuade Sandoz not to make it too expensive but I think it will be quite expensive. Up until now supplies have been free.

Kennedy: The simple effect of having a huge reduction in the number of patients with failed transplants having to return to dialysis will improve things enormously.

J. Feehally (Manchester Royal Infirmary): Could Prof Calne comment on any evidence that the use of cyclosporin A may be associated with an excess incidence of lymphoma or other lymphoproliferative disease?

Calne: Every immunosuppressive drug increases the incidence of all kinds of cancer but particularly lymphomata. When cyclosporin A was first used it was used in conjunction with other drugs and it was not realised how powerful it was. The development of lymphomata has been particularly common in heart transplant patients treated by conventional immunosuppression and there is no doubt that if patients are given too much immunosuppression lymphomata, probably virus-induced will develop. The virus that has been most implicated is the EB virus.

Since our initial experience with this drug, we have been very careful with the dosage. We have transplanted more than 100 patients since the report of the lymphomata without another lymphoma. In the multicentre trial, more than 100 patients were treated with cyclosporin A without developing lymphomata. So I do not think there is any evidence that cyclosporin A *per se* causes lymphomata. Cyclosporin A is a powerful immunosuppressant. If the patient is over-immunosuppressed T-cell function is completely paralysed and oncogenic viruses will produce lymphomata. But the same is true for any kind of immunosuppression.

R. Bailey (Royal Berkshire Hospital): If after donation a live donor's kidney actually failed, could that donor be considered for a transplant himself and how would it affect his prognosis?

Calne: I do not think this has ever happened, or if it has I have not heard of it.

   If such a situation arose then the patient would be no different from any other requiring a transplant.

H. Holder (Unicare Medical Services): Patients going home on CAPD now normally go home between 10 and 14 days after the catheter implant. Is that long enough to train a patient in the importance of sterile techniques during their exchanges at home?

   Secondly, how frequently are line changes performed at Manchester?

R. Gokal: 10 or 14 days is probably adequate for teaching patients the exchange procedure. But that is based on the assumption that a staff nurse or a sister is teaching all the time and that the patients are really put through a very intensive training programme for about 10 days.

   In Manchester we allow them home for a couple of days and bring them back in again during the training period and see how they have progressed at home. Our home CAPD sister visits them as well. The short period of training is adequate in terms of the technique and the expertise that they acquire, together with the knowledge of the complications.

   They may find it difficult to adjust psychologically to the technique and the dialysis life. Home haemodialysis patients have a training time of anything from 10 to 12 weeks and they have a much longer time to adjust to a new way of life. This is not the case for patients on CAPD. A fair number of problems that arise early on are related to this and that is where the home CAPD sister comes in. There is always a close liaison and back up and it can be done.

   Manufacturers currently recommend line changes every 4 weeks because they cannot guarantee the connections beyond that time. We need better catheters and connectors to extend the time interval.

   The alternative would be not to have a connecting set but to have a 1 m long catheter and do away with a set change altogether.

F. M. Parsons (Leeds General Infirmary): Bergström and his colleagues' original article on sequential ultrafiltration has not really been popularized as it should be. Initially, they ultrafiltered only.

When they commenced dialysis, unlike the vast majority of units in Europe, they used a sodium concentration in their dialysis fluid in excess of 140 mmol/l. They also used acetate. There are now quite a number of reports that one can ultrafilter almost at the same rate as they advocated using initial sodium concentrations in dialysis fluid of 145–150 mmol/l; after 2 hours of dialysis the sodium concentration can be gradually reduced to more conventional levels. I do not believe a single word of Bergström's theory on sequential ultrafiltration. Perhaps Dr Walls could comment.

J. Walls: We have been used to Dr Parsons's sceptical remarks for many years!

Experience shows that, without a shadow of doubt, in the patient with acute pulmonary oedema, isolated ultrafiltration without diffusion is a very valuable technique. I am well aware of the point about the increase in the dialysis fluid sodium concentrations. There is also the work from Chen and colleagues (1980) where the sodium concentration was increased to over 150 mmol/l. These studies, as far as I am aware, were relatively short-term, and one is constantly concerned about the effects of high sodium concentrations in dialysis fluid on the longterm management of hypertension in chronic renal failure. I am not aware of any study that has gone on for, say, 12 months, looking at this aspect. These studies were of individual dialyses on large numbers of patients.

Parsons: Yesterday I demanded from the Department of Health, an answer within a month to the staffing problems of CAPD. I asked how are we going to get it to work. Perhaps I am the only person present of the original working party that established intermittent dialysis in the 1960s. I said in that working party that renal physicians did not stand a chance of getting money from regional hospital boards for there was at most only one renal physician per region. The Department recalled the working party within 2 weeks and gave us the money, so it can be done.

I was most impressed with Dr Gokal's observations about the staff loading required for establishing a CAPD unit and congratulate him on his observations. But I hope that I have been able to stress the problems that he presented so well regarding funding the staff. This has got to come from central government for we will not get it from regional authorities.

It was done in the 1960s and I still stick to my timetable of 4 weeks despite the fact that the DHSS may take a week off for Easter!

G. Pincherle (DHSS): I am not aware that Dr Parsons has made any official request to the central department. If and when we receive one it will be considered, but it is not the policy of this government to make central money available that is earmarked for any specific initiative in any field. The policy is to make global sums available to regional health authorities who will then allocate it in the light of priorities.

R. Banks (Southmead Hospital): None of us who are involved in CAPD programmes would ever like to see this become a truly second class treatment programme for patients in renal failure. But in the real world we are all of us accepting patients on to our programmes who are undoubtedly at a much higher risk than those previously accepted for haemodialysis. I think particularly of patients with ischaemic heart disease and with systemic disease. Should we not face up to that and stop trying to compare our results all the time with those of haemodialysis?

Gokal: Dr Walls presented a slide showing that haemodialysis is the gold standard. If a new treatment becomes available there has to be something by which we can gauge that treatment. The only standard that is available now is home haemodialysis. In the good units I do not think there is all that much difference in the technique dropout rate between home haemodialysis and home CAPD. There is a difference but it is not all that marked.

But yes, we live in a real world, and although these are the sort of ideal standards that one would like to have, I am putting a lot of patients who are high risk on to CAPD because if I do not do that there is no treatment at all. And it is a matter of life and death in a lot of instances in an area where dialysis facilities are really very low. The Manchester Area is probably at the bottom of the UK league and the UK is at the bottom of the European league, so it is obvious how far behind we are.

W. Cattell (St Bartholomew's Hospital): This is a multi-disciplinary meeting with many nurses, patients and so on participating. It would be unfortunate if they went away with the feeling that HLA typing is now irrelevant in transplantation. I am perfectly aware that there is considerable discussion around the world. Mr Wood, I know, has strong personal feelings on it. But I think even he would agree that there is no universal agreement on dismissing HLA typing. It may well be mixed up with the centre effect and until such time as we have had more time to look at that it would be foolish to forget about it.

My immediate question is that we are now all aware of the enhancing effect of pre-transfusion in terms of graft survival. However, the price we pay is that if we transfuse patients we run the risk of sensitization with the development of antibodies. I am very attracted by the policy which I understand operates in Leiden in which they deliberately transfuse one unit, and one unit only, of fresh blood which they believe to be sufficient to induce the protective effect. Thereafter, if for clinical reasons they have to transfuse, they use lymphocyte-free blood, produced I gather by filtration processes.

Would Mr Wood go along with this concept or has he any observations to make on it.

R. F. M. Wood: To take Dr Cattell's first point. I do not think it would be sad if people went away from this meeting thinking that HLA-A and HLA-B typing did not have a tremendous amount to offer, certainly to the recipients of first cadaver grafts. There is no evidence that it really is of particular value. The collaborative study in the USA recently did show that there was no statistically significant advantage from HLA-A and HLA-B matching. All that HLA-A and HLA-B matching does in first transplants is to reduce the incidence of cytotoxic antibody formation should the graft fail. But it is of no other great benefit. It is now very difficult to get decent HLA-A and HLA-B matches. If we look at the UK transplant figures over the years, the number of patients who have had a 3- or 4-antigen match is very very small, and most patients are in fact being transplanted with mismatched kidneys anyway. I do not think that there is any prospect of improving HLA-A and HLA-B matching. Nor do I think that it is worth the effort. Some people have shown, like the Newcastle Group, that matching for the B locus is of some advantage, but really it is much better to put our efforts into HLA-DR matching, and I think that that is likely to be of considerably greater benefit.

When it comes to second transplants HLA-A and HLA-B matching is of importance. In the group of patients that I talked about who had the broadly reactive antibodies that reacted with CLL cells, there is good evidence that the only hope of transplantation is to get a kidney that is both HLA-A and HLA-B matched and is also HLA-DR matched. That is of some importance.

Dr Cattell's second point was on blood transfusion. The group in Leiden have shown that one transfusion at the time of operation is effective. There is a study from Oxford (Williams *et al.*, 1980) which also showed that transfusion at the time of operation was effective in enhancing graft survival. Some units have gone a little bit overboard in their elective transfusion policy and they have been giving people up to six units of whole blood. There is clear evidence that the more blood that is given, the higher the risk of sensitization. I think people should look at the number of transfusions they are giving and not over-transfuse patients. That is important.

Dr Cattell also mentioned the Leiden results using lymphocyte-free blood. There is very conflicting evidence about what type of blood should be used; whether it should be frozen, washed red cells, or some other type. There is evidence now that things like platelets perhaps may be particularly important, and perhaps even a transfusion of platelets might be the answer. There has been a lot of work done by Hans Jekkel and the group in Maastricht on trying to identify which bit of the blood is particularly important, but at the moment we still don't know as far as human results are concerned.

P. F. Williams (Western General Hospital): What are Mr Wood's views on donor-specific transfusion for living related donors?

Wood: The evidence from the United States is that donor-specific trans-fusion is of value. What is interesting is that cyclosporin A is known to inhibit antibody production. One of the exciting developments that we may see is the combination of using donor-specific transfusion and cyclosporin A in combination to prevent the antibody formation, but hopefully still to produce the enhancing effect.

But I think there is good evidence to support donor-specific blood trans-fusion in living related donors.

R. Banks (Southmead Hospital): Has Dr Dobbie any further information on the changes he has shown very nicely on electron microscope? Are they reversible at all, and can this be of practical significance. Presumably the loss of ultrafiltration that occurs in some people on CAPD after a while might be reversible if they are switched over to haemodialysis and the peri-toneum allowed to restructure.

J. Dobbie: As yet I cannot give a complete answer to this. I could mention some miscellaneous facts that we have observed so far. The mesothelium is extremely delicate and is stripped off by exposure to even normal saline. Dialysis fluid is certainly not just normal saline and its pH is quite acid.

This can be demonstrated simply in the experimental animal by exposing a piece of caecum without touching it and then either drying it or dropping on saline or dialysis fluid. The mesothelium comes off.

So it may well be, and as yet we cannot say, that once dialysis starts the patients no longer have any mesothelium and that they dialyse through the basal lamina in the submesothelial tissues. I would not be surprised if that occurs in most patients. The dialysis fluid probably comes into equilibrium with the fluid-containing mucopolysaccharides of the subserosa, and people dialyse through this. I do not think the mesothelium offers much in the way of a barrier. But these are as yet unsupported speculations.

The mesothelium is very delicate and probably dialysis takes place despite its absence.

P. Little (National Federation of Kidney Patients' Associations): Does what Mr Wood said about HLA-DR typing in cadaver transplantation also apply to live donor transplants, and how does that tie in with the possible significance of HLA-B matching? Would he exclude someone from having a live donor or cadaver transplant on the basis of a HLA-B mismatch if there was a good HLA-DR match.

Wood: I do not think there is really enough information about the effect of HLA-DR matching donor transplants. The point about live donors is that there is the time to do traditional D locus matching using MLC and that is probably more important.

The second point concerned the relative importance of HLA-B and HLA-DR matching. We are faced constantly with a clinical situation in which a kidney comes up and we need to decide who is the best match. I think programmes should now be organized on the basis of HLA-DR matching and I think it is quite logical on the evidence that has been produced to go for a match on the B locus as well. I am not trying to advocate a policy of disregarding tissue matching. It is important and one should go for the best match one can get. But it is a question of which priority to put first. I do not think that the use of HLA-A and HLA-B as an initial sorting code is tenable any longer.

I think HLA-DR should be used as the initial sorting code.

Kennedy: We have had a very full and varied session.

References

Chen, W-T., Ing, T. S., Daugirdas, J. T., Humayun, H. M., Brescia, D. J., Gandhi, V. C., Hano, J. E. and Kheirbek, A. O. (1980). Hydrostatic ultrafiltration during haemodialysis using decreasing sodium dialysate. *Artif. Organs,* **4,** 187

Williams, K. A., French, M. E., Ting, A., Oliver, D. and Morris, P. J. (1980). Preoperative blood-transfusions improve cadaveric renal-allograft survival in non-transfused recipients. *Lancet,* **1,** 1104

SESSION FOUR

Psychological, Social and Ethical Aspects
Chairman:
W. Cattell

Chairman's Introduction
W. Cattell

Let me begin by recalling that in the middle sixties Shaldon pioneered in Britain the development of self-supervised home dialysis. This was shown to be immensely successful and has been the mainstay of haemodialysis in the United Kingdom ever since.

At that time, a sort of euphoria came over the clinicians of Britain as they really did believe that this was the answer to everything, and it was with no little temerity that in 1970 at the EDTA Meeting in Barcelona we presented a paper (Gordon and Cattell, 1970) which challenged the basis for this euphoria about home dialysis. Our concern was that while this was cost-effective and successful, it did make immense demands on the patient and on the patient's family—social, psychological and economic demands. I think that in fairness the paper was well received, and since that time most of us involved in renal replacement in the United Kingdom have been intensely aware of the demands made not just on our patients, but on our patients' families, on the staff, the dedicated nurses, technicians and so on. While we are concerned with the inadequacies of the facilities that we have which prevent us from treating all the patients we would like, it is essential that at all times we do not lose sight of the welfare of those people whom we already have on treatment, the patients of today, and of our staff.

It is my personal belief that a multidisciplinary symposium such as this would be wholly incomplete if there were not some opportunity to discuss just this sort of thing.

The title of the symposium in Stirling was 'Living with Renal Failure' and the title of this one is 'Who Cares?'. I would submit that the people who really know about living with renal failure and the people who really care

are the patients, the patients' families, and those staff who are intimately and daily in contact with the patients.

It is therefore a considerable pleasure for me to introduce this session, which in some ways may be one of the most important of the whole symposium.

16

Social and psychological issues of end-stage renal failure
J. Auer

16.1   INTRODUCTION

There are many studies of the problems and stresses experienced by haemodialysis patients and their families, and therefore this paper attempts to consider some of the new, along with the well documented areas.

The rapid growth of continuous ambulatory peritoneal dialysis (CAPD)
programmes has produced new types of problems amongst patients' families,
and their staff. One aim of this presentation is to compare and constrast the
social and psychological effects of haemodialysis and CAPD at different
stages, eventually leading to rehabilitation on home treatment. These
effects and their impact on adjustment depend above all on the personality
of the patient, his strengths and weaknesses and the quality of support
available from the family and the hospital team. While there are many
similarities in the stresses on patients, there are very diverse responses,
which demand great understanding and flexibility from those involved in
treatment.

16.2   PRE-DIALYSIS ASSESSMENT AND ADJUSTMENT

The patient attending a pre-dialysis clinic is in a state of transition,
characterized by uncertainties, fears and anticipation of loss. The chief
problems are:

Fear of death – doubts about life expectancy,
Fear of the unknown – fantasies about treatment,
Doubts about the future – employment and finances,
Relationship problems due to effects of illness,
   e.g. irritability, impaired concentration, fatigue, loss of libido, guilt,
   fear of dependence, role reversal,
'Unfinished business' – unresolved personal matters
   which impede adjustment,
Denial – inability to accept the need for treatment.

The pre-dialysis period offers a chance for full assessment of the patient,
especially his attitudes to his situation. Some fears and fantasies can be dispelled, for example a surprising number believe that dialysis can prolong
life for a short time only. Many others believe that the treatment is a very
painful process. Although CAPD is a simple system to describe, it can give
rise to misconceptions. For instance a distressed lady, who had been offered
the treatment and shown a 2 litre bag, confessed tearfully that she was
afraid that her bladder would not hold that amount for 4 hours. At this
stage patients may benefit from talking to somebody already established
satisfactorily on haemodialysis or CAPD.

The pro's and con's of haemodialysis and CAPD can be discussed so that
the patient's employment, personality and lifestyle may be taken into con-

sideration before a final choice of treatment is made. Discussion with the spouse and family allows anxieties to be ventilated and some can be dispelled. In addition, the quality of support required and previous patterns of interaction can be assessed.

Wherever possible, every effort to maintain employment should be encouraged even if a change to lighter or part-time work is needed. There is no doubt that those who continue working before dialysis is commenced are those who tend to do so on dialysis and after transplantation, those who give up work, lose motivation, confidence and self-esteem.

Anxiety and depression are often unexpressed, but are usually present. Uraemia and the side-effects of anti-hypertensive drugs (Whitlock and Evans, 1978) may be partly responsible, but much stress derives from uncertainty, helplessness, and loss of the ability to control events. Reassurance and information may enable a degree of planning to mitigate this. Fatigue, irritability and guilt have often made the patient hard to live with, and relationships may be under strain. A number of men already suffering from loss of libido have never connected this with their illness, and are relieved to learn that this is a symptom of the disease, which is less damaging to their sexual self-esteem. Partners too are relieved, having convinced themselves that they had competition, or were losing their attractiveness.

Unresolved personal stresses often come into sharp focus when facing renal failure. Three of our patients became preoccupied with getting divorced in order to marry longstanding co-habitees, and legitimize children. Others produce and work-through grief over past bereavements. Only when such 'unfinished' business is resolved can the patient's energies be turned to tackling the future.

Denial serves a useful purpose in coping with anxiety while adjustment progresses (Short and Wilson, 1969). As such, it need only be challenged if it is a serious threat to health, for instance in gross dietary abuse or repeated failure to attend clinics. Denial in the spouse can equally serve the interests of the patient, or become dysfunctional, due to unrealistic expectations of capabilities. It may also lead to a blocking of communication about needs and feelings.

16.2.1 Starting haemodialysis

The patient starting haemodialysis after months, or even years in a pre-dialysis clinic, usually follows a typical pattern of response. Initially anxiety occurs, followed by a euphoric sense of relief due to the benefits of treatment, with the welcome discovery that the experience is less unpleasant than expected. It is usually after 2–6 weeks that a depressive reaction ensues. This may show itself in a flippant attitude, demanding behaviour, aggression and irritability, or apathy and disinterest. All these represent attempts by the patient to cope with stress. A few patients continue to use denial and test out the limitations of their new circumstances by ignoring diet and fluid restrictions or trying to miss a dialysis. Patients who feel guilt due to adverse effects on spouse and family may be resentful and truculent in the unit. While all such reactions present exasperating problems for the nursing staff, it is perhaps the 'model patient' who should arouse most suspicion. Such patients are often either repressing their feelings excessively, or exhibiting their frustrations at home. A patient referred recently because of aggression and miserable behaviour on dialysis explained that this enabled him to be pleasant to his family on returning home.

During the long hospital training, the patient usually forms strong and supportive relationships with both staff and other patients, and begins to feel one of a special and exclusive community

16.2.2 Starting CAPD

An increasing number of patients start CAPD with little or no preparation in a pre-dialysis clinic. Acute presentation of chronic renal failure is for many reasons more likely to be treated by CAPD. In these cases the patient is given no time either for anxiety or adjustment, and is often in a numbed or bewildered state for the first few days. Since training time is short, most patients can and do come to a quick superficial acceptance of the situation. Signs that they are not able to do so include unwillingness or slowness to learn exchange technique and complaints that they are being rushed. They may be given different instructions by different nurses which can increase confusion. If anxiety and giddiness develop on mobilization careful investigation is required since symptoms of postural hypotension often mimic anxiety attacks.

16.3 RETURNING HOME

16.3.1 Initial period of haemodialysis

When the healthy spouse attends for training, the patient becomes very aware of imminent separation from the unit. The healthy spouse is often lacking in confidence and both husband and wife need much understanding from staff. Patients are often irritable and domineering towards a timid and slow learning spouse, especially if the patient is the dominant partner. (Strelzer *et al.*, 1976). Many healthy spouses feel that their partner receives all the unit's sympathy and attention, while their own needs and predicament have received little recognition.

Returning home with the machine is always an anxious time for the couple. However proficient they have become, it is one thing to have trained help on hand, and quite another to be miles from the unit. The patient often misses the hospital community, particularly the staff and fellow patients, who have become his friends during the crisis of his illness. Bonds formed during periods of vulnerability are particularly strong. Some therefore need careful weaning from the unit, and may at first telephone frequently with trivial complaints. The position is better for those patients who have maintained outside interests and especially employment. For them dialysis has never become the sole focus of life.

16.3.2 Initial period of CAPD

The CAPD patient generally shows less anxiety about returning home, and has had less time to become part of the hospital unit community. In many cases however, the lack of time for adjustment catches up with the patient, and he may become depressed, self-neglectful and an immediate candidate for peritonitis, or perhaps so obsessional about technique that he isolates himself at home, taking little advantage of the potential freedom offered by the treatment. It may be many months before he gains enough confidence to try an exchange away from home. In the case of elderly patients it is often the spouse or family who show anxiety by pressing for readmission.

16.3.3 Longterm

With high unemployment, even patients who have missed little work through illness, tend to be among the first to be made redundant, when the workforce is reduced. It can be helpful to register the patient as disabled because of the statutory duty of employers to have a percentage of disabled employees, but renal patients naturally dislike the implied stigma. With unemployment come greater financial problems and further loss of self-esteem. Marriages are put under increased strain, especially when the wife becomes the only breadwinner, as well as the dialysis helper.

The break from routine afforded by a holiday presents problems for the haemodialysis patient, spouse and family, both from the treatment and financial point of view. Patients associations both local and national are fortunately making more and more holiday facilities available, thus not only giving the healthy spouse a respite from the task of dialysis, but relieving the guilt of the patient, whose situation otherwise denies his family a normal pleasure. The occasional relief of spouses is necessary when they are ill or overstressed. Their absence could be met by local minimum care units, but unfortunately there are as yet too few of these. Hopefully their number will increase in the future.

Marital problems, directly or indirectly related to illness and treatment, frequently arise after a couple have apparently been settled on home dialysis for a long period. Direct causes include loss of libido in the patient, leading to lack of affectionate contact and communication, the inability to start, or add to, a family, fatigue and irritability of the patient, and the stress and time involved in treatment. Indirect causes include social isolation, especially among young people on CAPD, financial difficulties and behaviour problems with children, who suffer as a result of their parents' preoccupation with treatment, leaving little time or energy to spare (Mass and de Nour, 1975).

Young unmarried CAPD patients have difficulty in forming relationships (Auer, 1981). The catheter, bag, and abdominal distension make them feel unattractive to the opposite sex. This leads to self-neglect, smart clothing is abandoned and loss of confidence is evident. These difficulties are comparable in many respects with those of patients with stomas. One 20-year-old described his position in these words, 'What young girl wants a boyfriend who carries around a plastic bag like an incontinent old man!'. Older CAPD patients are less concerned with self-image and marriages and, in spite of more reported sexual difficulties, exhibit less tension. Role changes are rare, partly because the spouse is not involved in treatment.

16.4 DEPRESSION AND ANXIETY IN HAEMODIALYSIS AND CAPD PATIENTS

Depression and anxiety levels in both patients and spouses tend to be higher than in the general population. Even where a marriage is severely strained, the guilt and practical difficulties associated with leaving a sick partner frequently prevent a separation, which might have been the outcome but for the illness.

When a patient fails to achieve a satisfactory longterm adjustment, it is more common for anxiety to be the most prominent psychological problem in the haemodialysis patient, and depression in the CAPD patient, although a combination is commonly found.

16.5 EFFECTS OF SUCCESSFUL TRANSPLANTATION

Many successful transplant patients have practical and psychological difficulties in adjusting to 'normal' life. Those who had previously given up work while on dialysis, often delay looking for re-employment. There is uncertainty about the graft and its future, fears of damaging the kidney or of exposure to infection, but primarily a fear of giving up the invalid role and having to compete once more on 'equal' terms (Salmons, 1980).

16.5.1 Work potential

Medical staff may declare the patient fit for work, but attach provisos, which make the offer of a job unlikely. Many patients seeking work post-transplant, with a clean bill of health find that prospective employers see their 'fitness' as either temporary or partial, and will not risk offering a job. The DHSS, however, rules that such a patient is fit, and many find themselves with a suddenly reduced income, on unemployment benefit. Attendance allowance and invalidity benefit are no longer payable, and mobility allowance may also be lost. Some families therefore end up some £30-40 per week worse off than when the patient was on haemodialysis. Retraining through the Disablement Resettlement Officer is sometimes possible, but sadly many are still unable to get work afterwards.

16.5.2 Emotional problems

Patients who develop severe acne, hirsutism, or grossly cushingoid features on steroid therapy, may be very disturbed by their altered self-image. They can lose the confidence necessary for the pursuit of everyday life. Other side-effects of steroids such as depression, hypomanic behaviour, and emotional lability are severely disabling in some cases.

16.5.3 Marital problems

These fall into two main categories. The first is pre-existing disharmony, which had become of secondary importance during the crisis of renal failure and treatment by dialysis. Once the patient is comparatively fit, such discord may resume its former prominence, and lead to marital breakdown.

The other common problem is sexual difficulty, and this may occur in patient or spouse. A few patients previously potent become impotent after transplantation. Some, previously lacking in libido, expected transplantation to restore full function, and are dismayed if this doesn't occur. Some patients who regain libido find that their partner, following a long period of sexual inactivity, has lost potency or interest. Some spouses have assumed a nursing or parental role towards the dialysis patient, and cannot easily switch back to being a lover.

While the majority of transplant patients make a satisfactory adjustment and reap the full benefits of renewed health, a disturbingly large minority cannot adjust, either because of external or internal problems.

16.6 SEXUAL PROBLEMS

A common pattern following loss of libido is:

(1) Decrease of affectionate contact,
(2) Decrease in verbal expression of feelings,
(3) Communication becomes very limited, with large taboo areas.

16.6.1 Counselling

Counselling cannot restore libido or potency where the cause of the problem is largely physical, but it can help to keep the relationship alive. Expression of affection both verbal and through touch can be encouraged, so that both partners feel valued. Communication of needs and feelings may be gradually increased. A female spouse, for example, may have been afraid to ask her partner for manual or oral stimulation. Female patients often describe their partners as 'very patient, very undemanding'. In such cases the wife who encourages intercourse despite her lack of libido, and expresses pleasure in her husband's attentions, is able to enhance the relationship.

A further aim of counselling is to give practical advice. Residual libido is most often present in the early morning, when natural hormone levels are at their highest and libido-suppressing drug levels are at their lowest. Two couples counselled recently have achieved successful intercourse with this advice. In both cases the frustrated wife had believed her husband impotent for over a year, and had resorted to taking sleeping pills at night. Neither had been wakeable, let alone physically arouseable, in the early morning. It is sad that due to loss of communication, these couples had not solved the difficulty themselves.

16.6.2 Myths and fears

Myths and fears about the dangers of intercourse with CAPD can be discussed, and alternative positions suggested where appropriate. Changed body-image, leading to loss of confidence, can best be helped by talking to the couple together. Most spouses do not find the catheter offputting, but most patients believe it is until reassured otherwise. Self-image is usually reflected in the manner of dress. A number of patients on CAPD abandon any attempt to look attractive.

The CAPD sister is normally best placed to pick up the patients' spoken or unspoken messages about himself, and to offer advice and counselling.

16.7 NEW ETHICAL PROBLEMS WITH THE INTRODUCTION OF CAPD

The introductions of CAPD has now made it possible to treat a number of patients previously excluded from most programmes. These include the elderly, diabetics, those with cardiovascular disease, some with access problems and those with multiple medical problems. Many of these patients present acutely, giving little or no time for either full assessment or enquiries into social circumstances before treatment commences. In some instances, treatment cannot prolong life for more than 6–12 months because of underlying disease, such as amyloid or myeloma. A fair proportion of that time will be spent on learning the technique of CAPD, particularly as training of patients falling into these categories usually takes longer than average. Two paraplegics in their mid-fifties, one with severe IHD and the other with widespread amyloid, were trained for CAPD. The first was in hospital for 3 months and lived for 2 weeks at home, the second was in hospital for 4 months before dying from amyloidosis.

If the patients complete training there may be frequent readmissions due either to peritonitis or other medical problems. Relatives of elderly or sick patients carry a great burden of care, especially if the patient is widowed or living alone.

Most of us have had experience of the patient, who, after rational and realistic consideration, wants to stop treatment. We know the stress and guilt felt by the families, and indeed by the staff of the unit when a patient takes this decision. This causes a dilemma. Should the treatment have been started in the first place, and who should be involved in making the final decision? Occasionaly it is put to the family that an elderly patient could be kept alive by CAPD for a year or more, but would need constant help and supervision. The family feel that they are being asked 'How much do you care?'. They probably have no idea of the realities of doing 4-hourly exchanges, nor of the quality of life being offered. If they decline, however, they carry a huge burden of guilt. I am convinced that no family should be made to feel that they have connived at the death of a relative.

As in the case of living related transplant donors, the offer to help in undertaking CAPD for an elderly relative should come from the family unprompted, and, preferably, should survive active discouragement It is even harder to involve a patient, depressed, uraemic, and ignorant of what is really involved, with making a rational choice, before treatment starts.

In two recent cases, the patients, both women approaching 70, were reluctant to be treated. However, after the team had considered their good quality of life before the development of renal failure, and their family circumstances they were persuaded to accept treatment. Both are thriving, one having just returned from her second foreign holiday in 6 months.

Another recurrent dilemma is the patient who presents acutely, needing immediate treatment without proper assessment, who turns out to have almost insurmountable social or psychological problems.

Acute presentation correlates positively with increase in age and social or psychological problems. With CAPD, these groups can be treated, but rehabilitation is frequently lengthy and quality of life poor. When CAPD fails the patient is usually transferred to haemodialysis, since the commitment to treatment is generally non-specific. As a result home dialysis training programmes for suitable patients risk becoming blocked by these failed CAPD patients for whom home dialysis is usually impossible for medical and social reasons.

16.8   CONCLUSIONS

For the first time in many years, dialysis programmes are feeling the impact of a new approach to treatment in CAPD. This presents both opportunities and dilemmas, not least in making treatment available for the elderly and those with social problems incompatible with haemodialysis. The possibilities cannot yet be assessed, because we need to know more about the longterm effects. Whatever treatment is chosen, it can be seen that there is a need to maintain awareness of the social and psychological effects upon patients and their families, through constant reassessment. There should be a flexible approach to individual needs, and, if necessary, appropriate counselling to achieve the best possible rehabilitation for each patient.

In our enthusiasm for new treatment methods, it is important not to lose sight of the central aim of the renal unit team, which is, and should remain, to ensure good quality of life for our patients.

References

Auer, J. (1981). Quality of life on CAPD, related to sex and age-group: a comparison with haemodialysis. *Proc. Eur. Dial. Transplant Nursing Assoc.*, **9**, 204

Mass, M. and de-Nour, A. K. (1975). Reactions of families to chronic hemodialysis. *Psychother. Psychosom.*, **26**, 20

Salmons, P. H. (1980). Psychosocial aspects of chronic renal failure. *Br. J. Hosp. Med.*, **23**, 617

Short, M. J. and Wilson, W. P. (1969). Roles of denial in chronic hemodialysis. *Arch. Gen. Psychiatry*, **20**, 433

Streltzer, J., Finkelstein, F., Feigenbaum, R. M., Kitson, J. and Cohen, G. L. (1976). The spouse's role in home hemodialysis. *Arch. Gen. Psychiatry,* **33**, 55

Whitlock, F. A. and Evans, L. E. J. (1978). Drugs and depression. *Drugs,* **15**, 53

17

Stress amongst staff in the renal unit
E. A. Winder

17.1 INTRODUCTION

It is highly unlikely that anyone involved in any aspect of the care of renal patients is not aware that stress exists, not only amongst the patients themselves, but amongst the staff as well.

The stresses, in my opinion, are very little different for the doctor or the nurse. However, they may be perceived differently and therefore have different effects. Although some of us definitely earn less than others within the renal team, very few (in the United Kingdom anyway), make a fortune out of it. This implies that we must have wanted to get involved in this field of medicine for reasons other than making money. I am never quite sure why junior hospital doctors choose nephrology, but it is ironic that the very motive which inspires so many nurses to enter the renal field, the desire to have a meaningful ongoing relationship with the patient, so often proves to be the source of greatest emotional stress.

17.2   SYMPTOMS AND RESULTS OF STRESS

Stress amongst nurses working in high dependency areas is well documented. 'Burnout', as our American cousins call it, can occur when a staff member feels that despite all she is doing (and she often feels that she is the only one doing it) neither her patient nor her seniors appreciate her work. Furthermore, her patients are not getting better. The symptoms of 'burnout' are frighteningly recognizable: (1) physical and emotional exhaustion, irritability; (2) stress-related illnesses such as colds, headaches, stomach ailments and excessive complaining; and (3) rigidity in decision making, over-eating and chronic fatigue.

Manifestations of stress can be seen in dissension amongst different levels of staff. This gives rise to a loss of morale and, finally, to nurses leaving the unit. The reasons for leaving are twofold:

(1)   They can earn precisely the same peanuts working in another area of the hospital or community where the patients are just as deserving of nursing time and where the nurses will not be expected to work overtime. There the pace of work is such that they are able to give proper nursing care and, at the end of a shift, they can go off duty and feel that they have not only done a good day's work but are alive and awake enough to cook their husband's supper.

(2)   The second reason applies to fewer nurses, but sadly the more committed and professionally aware. If a staff nurse stays in nephrology long enough, and is good enough, she may eventually get a job as a sister. If she stays a sister long enough, she may just be lucky enough to be in the right place at the right time to get one of the few renal nursing officer posts. After that, if she wants to develop her career, she is at present forced to leave her specialist career behind her and become a non-clinical nurse administrator, or go into nursing education.

So apart from the love of the job (including all the stress and anxiety that goes with it) there is not much incentive for staff to stay on as a specialist in renal nursing. Now that is a very important point, because it does not matter how famous a hospital or renal unit may be. It does not matter how many transplants a particular surgeon may do in a year nor does it matter how good the standard of medicine is if there are not enough nurses to dialyse the patients and nurse the transplants. So it is in the interests of all who care about the future of nephrology in this country to look at ways in which at least some of the stress to staff can be reduced. The incentives should also be increased.

17.3 THE ROLE OF THE RENAL UNIT MANAGER

There are, of course, many ways in which the renal unit manager can help. It is vitally important that the unit manager should be the following:

(1) An expert clinical renal nurse so that she is able to lead the nursing team effectively. A purely managerial or administrative nursing officer to a renal unit, is in my opinion, a complete waste of time for she will not be able to manage the people or the situations if she has no understanding of them. And a junior nurse (or even a senior nurse for that matter) who has just done a lousy dialysis on a well loved patient feels pretty bad. It is worth remembering that there is probably no other area of nursing where it is so easy to render your patient moribund or just give them yet another rotten day. Admittedly giving people a bad dialysis is totally avoidable – but its amazing how often it happens even in the best planned units.

(2) Seen to have a liberal attitude to off-duty, holiday requests, study leave and to ensure that overtime and on-call payments are made without fuss.

(3) Capable of making sure that the renal ward nurses attend transplant out-patient clinics, and that the dialysis nurses change frequently from working in the maintenance dialysis unit to doing the acute renal failure dialyses in the intensive care units. This serves to remind nurses that there is no single treatment of choice for our patients and that if CAPD fails, haemodialysis or transplantation is available, or if the transplant fails, hospital dialysis will be offered until a further transplant can be arranged. Admittedly, we are lucky to have all five treatments available within our unit.

(4) Able to arrange, encourage and provide financial assistance for nurses to visit other centres or attend meetings, where they can share their experiences. This may all sound very obvious but I have visited more than one maintenance dialysis unit which refers patients to other centres for transplantation where no-one, including the dialysis nurses themselves, have ever thought to arrange a visit to the transplant centre.

17.4 DEFUSING THE SITUATION

Stress obviously increases as workload increases, and I do not believe my own unit at Guy's is unique in doing 179% more dialyses now than in 1974 but with only a 33% increase in nurses. Everyone is working at near crisis point and consequently, 'nursing care' goes out of the window. This causes lack of job satisfaction for the nurses and presumable 'burnout'. Nurses are sceptical about whether they should come and work with us or choose something easier. This means that staff vacancies are difficult to fill and consequently the few that do come have to work that bit harder. I am sure that at Guy's one of the major factors which has kept us all going is that we are a very closely knit and collaborative team, and, without realizing it, we have been doing one of the things which is supposed to reduce the effects of 'burnout'. This is called PSD, programmed staff defusing, and we do it at our weekly unit meeting. This was ostensibly set up to discuss the patient's problems in a truly multidisciplinary way. Quite often, at our Monday meetings there are 40 people present these include as many of our nine sisters as possible, myself, the senior and junior medical staff, the dietician, social worker, home dialysis administrator, chief technician and transplant surgeon. In addition nurses from all areas of the unit and other interested parties also attend. This meeting gives us the chance to share information and keep the team informed. It also allows individuals, particularly the nurses, to express their opinions and air their views. It is often a long and exhausting meeting but I believe strongly that it has a therapeutic effect in allowing everyone to feel their voice can be heard.

The essence of effective collaboration in a health care team is the agreement of mutual aims and trust and respect for each others' competencies. Undoubtedly problems will arise if this collaboration is non-existent.

17.5 SUMMARY

In summary, to attract and then keep renal nurses, we need to:

(1) Provide education at grass roots level.
(2) Be kind to them.
(3) Provide a clinical career structure.
(4) Make them part of the renal team.

The frustrations of working in an under-financed National Health Service, which appears to give little or no priority to the plight of the renal patient, means that those of us who do care are working under constantly increasing pressure. Unless we are prepared to look after and support each other within the team, I believe we will fail to be able to support and look after our patients.

18

The patient's viewpoint
B. Pearmain, D. Benoliel, P. Little and R. Page

18.1 THE NATIONAL FEDERATION OF KIDNEY PATIENTS' ASSOCIATIONS

I would first like to outline the function of the National Federation of Kidney Patients' Associations. The organization was founded in October 1978, mainly to act as an information exchange for the growing number of voluntary patients' associations which were being formed at renal units throughout the country. Since then we have developed into the prime organization representing patients' views and we have established valuable links with the Department of Health up to Ministerial level. We have 33 member associations from every part of the country and our emphasis is on patient participation; our constitution requires that our executive committee consists of a majority of patients. Collectively we represent about 5000 patients and the total funds raised by our member associations runs into many hundreds of thousands of pounds each year. We are unique in that we are the only national organization in the country run by kidney patients for kidney patients.

The patient's view of the three modes of treatment will of course differ from those of other people because we are in the unique position of actually receiving and carrying out the treatment ourselves. All patients recognize and accept that we are the ones who are stuck with the problem and, where possible, we elect to have the treatment that will give us the least complications and the one that allows us to pursue the life style we want. Undoubtedly the successful transplant is the most popular goal sought by patients, particularly in the early days of treatment when any type of therapy seems fraught with difficulties. Nevertheless, it is quite suprising to many observers that a number of patients, when acquainted with some of the problems associated with transplantation, in particular rejection and its attendant psychological difficulties, steroid side-effects and disruption of an organized pattern of life through hospitalization, are content to forego the opportunity of a first or subsequent transplant.

Haemodialysis means different things to different patients but a patient's own attitude to this treatment has a great bearing on whether or not this form of treatment provides an acceptably high quality of life. My own experience, and that of many patients I have talked to, shows that a very positive stance must be taken towards haemodialysis to get the best out of it. I regard life on a machine in the same way as having a bad hand in a game of cards – play it the best way you can because there is a good chance you can win – but if you throw in your hand you throw away your chances and unlike a game of cards you do not get a second deal of life. Without wishing to sound flippant dialysis takes up about 20 hours a week of my life leaving another 148 hours to use to the best advantage. Having said this, no-one in their right mind would welcome the prospect of dialysis as a constant companion but neither would they welcome many other forms of longterm treatment of other ailments. Apart from the patient's own attitude, other vital factors help make haemodialysis easier. The staff of a renal unit play a great part in this by helping to guide the patient into a positive approach and of course there must be support and encouragement from the patient's family. My personal belief is that this is more likely to be successful with patients on home dialysis.

CAPD is of course still relatively new, but it is interesting to examine patients' attitudes to it. New patients I have talked to who have started immediately on this therapy are very happy with the results and are content to stay with it. I confess that 8 years ago when I first needed dialysis I think that I would have opted for CAPD if it had been offered, mainly because I did not like needles and the machine looked far too complex for me to master. Attitudes of many 'long service' patients I have talked to are very different, they regard CAPD as having a great nuisance factor in requiring four daily exchanges, 7 days a week, and they express concern at the risk of peritonitis. The attitude of patients to CAPD does seem to vary depending on the prevailing opinions of their unit staff but even so, many patients regard CAPD as the area where great progress is likely to be made during the next few years to make dialysis easier and better.

So much for the views of the patients; it is very interesting to examine how the public see us and the various forms of treatment. Whether we like it or not, the public's view of everything is greatly influenced by the media; very often their understanding or opinion of an unfamiliar subject is based almost exclusively on what is seen on TV, heard on radio or read in newspapers. I need only mention '*Panorama*' and transplants to prove that. It follows then that the public's view of kidney patients is based on media information, and it is quite remarkable how these opinions vary with the type of treatment.

The transplant patient is presented to the public as a success story; the transplant takes place, it is working and will do so for the next 30 years. The patient returns to normal life and goes back to work until old age carries him and the kidney into the grave. The rejections, the problems and the difficulties rarely get the same headlines; in my view this is absolutely right, because the public need to be encouraged to regard transplantation as the successful treatment that it is and so give it as much support as possible, particularly by carrying a kidney donor card.

Despite the relatively short time that CAPD has been available it is quite remarkable how much public knowledge there is of the treatment and how its value to patients is assessed. Again the media has generated a picture in the public's mind of a problem-free therapy and infers that it is available and suitable for everyone. In this instance I think a lot of credit for this image must go to the professional people who are really engaged in a type of product marketing programme. In itself this is not a bad thing because it is creating the all important positive approach, but there must be dangers in exaggerating the claims for the treatment that can raise false hopes in patients and produce major psychological problems when difficulties arise.

Haemodialysis on the other hand is treated quite differently by the media, and consequently tends to be regarded as the terror of the three possible therapies. The public are regularly told of the disadvantages of the treatment, and for some reason, patients who do not do well manage to find the headlines; rarely do the ones who cope well and live normal lives end up on the front pages. How many times have we read articles containing phrases like... 'suffers his 8 hour sessions twice every week' or... 'too weak to walk after her treatment' or... 'living in despair waiting for that phone call' (i.e. for a transplant). That sort of impression is as misleading to the public as saying that haemodialysis is great fun for everyone and presents no problems or restrictions. The true picture lies between the two extremes and the public need to be told what it is. I think everyone concerned with the welfare of kidney patients has a very real responsibility to present a more positive picture of haemodialysis as a treatment, not least because the greatest percentage of all patients start with haemodialysis and in the event of a rejected graft will return to it.

It should always be remembered that included amongst the public that has its views coloured by the media are general practitioners and doctors working in hospitals without renal units who are quite likely to make their judgements of whether or not to refer a patient to a renal unit in the light of what they have read or seen in the media. It is quite ridiculous for us to complain on the one hand about the non-referral of patients for treatment but on the other hand persuade those responsible for the referring that the treatment is worse than the disease! Also, future patients are part of the general public and it must be quite frightening for them to read of these untypical experiences in the media. They will be almost pre-conditioned to the idea that life is not going to be worth living and this makes the job of the renal unit staff even more difficult.

Finally I think our renal physicians deserve better support and encouragement. It must be very disheartening for a physician, having included a patient on his dialysis programme, often with great difficulty, to read newspaper reports that the patient is now 'suffering the agonies of thrice weekly dialysis' he must wonder why he bothered!

18.2 TRANSPLANTATION

What I have to say is a personal view, but my own experience has, I think, been augmented by that of the many other patients I have met in my work with Patients' Associations.

The response from my doctor when he heard I was to speak at the European Dialysis and Transplant Nurses Association Conference in Paris, 1981, was, 'Oh, no! I suppose you'll be saying that nobody ever explained anything to you!' So there is obviously an awareness on the part of the doctors that communication with patients could be improved. Now, as then, it is not my intention to indulge in 'doctor-bashing'.

It is to be hoped that patient-participation in renal conferences will become an established feature. Patients' associations have already done much to break down the 'them and us' attitudes unfortunately so prevalent in the past.

My renal disease was diagnosed in 1961 at a pre-employment medical. This demonstrates the value of this often maligned procedure. It is unusual today to have a routine medical examination as a young adult. One only goes to see a doctor when something is wrong. Preventive medicine has never been fashionable in Britain.

After much investigation I had a bladder-neck resection in 1961 and bilateral re-implantation of ureters in 1962. Continued deterioration of my kidney function led to a low-protein diet in 1969. Complete kidney failure occurred in 1970 and an arterio-venous fistula was constructed in my arm. A brief period of peritoneal dialysis was followed by training for haemodialysis early in 1971.

I dialysed at home for 8 years, working full-time in my profession of industrial pharmacy, and travelling abroad for holidays with portable machines of varying degrees of sophistication.

During this time I had a parathyroidectomy in 1975 and my first but unsuccessful transplant (accompanied by a life-threatening gastric haemorrhage) in 1977.

In 1979 I had my second transplant – so far successful. On that occasion I was a 'guinea-pig' for cyclosporin A which unfortunately did not work for me. I had 'epileptic' type fits and was unconscious for 3 days, but scraped through with a functioning kidney – but only just.

As you can see, transplantation can be dangerous and this brings me to the matter of better information for patients. Today, dialysis patients rightly hope for a quick and successful transplant but are, I feel, ill-prepared for the nature of the operation, the length of the subsequent recovery period, the likely rejection episodes and the risks involved in the immediate post-operative period. It is also not commonly known that long-term patient survival is better on haemodialysis than with a transplant. Far too often the decision by a patient to have a transplant is at best uninformed and at worst another stage in the drifting process – not really a decision at all. I would not want to exchange my present freedom for continuing dialysis, but some people might. The road is not always easy.

The benefits of transplantation are too obvious to mention but there are problems. The physical and emotional problems induced by high steroid doses initially are very distressing, and there are, of course, longterm side-effects of the immunosuppression, knowledge of which should not be kept from the potential recipient. I have felt that preparation for and advice about transplantation would have been very helpful to me and to my wife. I also have found adjusting to having a kidney, and its undoubted concomitant benefits, quite difficult. My experience is that having such a dramatic improvement in one's health can be just as psychologically devastating as having ill-health thrust upon one – only without the sympathy of friends and relatives, who cannot understand why you don't feel immediate joy and relief. This is not helped by the ignorance of most people who assume that all your problems are cured by a transplant. They have no idea that you may be walking a mental tightrope waiting for a rejection episode.

These feelings do pass with time. You begin to take good health for granted and start once more to complain of the little irritants of life – undoubtedly a good sign. Nevertheless, transplantation is not a cure. The saga of the disease goes o.i.

No matter how rapid the progress in treatment, everyone must work towards prevention of kidney disease. Unfortunately once treatments are available, particularly dramatic ones that catch the public imagination, some impetus for research into prevention is lost.

Telling people you have a transplanted kidney is, I find, very good 'public relations' for the cause of transplantation and often encourages people to carry donor cards. However, this is a personal attitude and not everyone will wish to disclose the fact that they have a transplant.

Membership of a patients association is of continuing value even when no longer on dialysis. I know that some dialysis patients feel that those of us with transplants are not patients any more – but we are! I feel it is helpful for patients with all forms of treatment to meet and discuss their problems and exchange information.

Doctors are now beginning to realize that there is no threat in patients banding together but that there are benefits to them also from this 'consumerism in medicine'. They find that better-informed and involved patients are able to understand their treatment better and make their doctors' lives easier.

I hope that I have managed to convey some of my feelings about life with dialysis and transplantation, and I do want to emphasize that, although I am a pharmacist and therefore have a medical and scientific training, my impression from talking to many patients of widely differing backgrounds is that all of us have had very similar doubts and fears about our illness.

18.3 HAEMODIALYSIS

It would be impossible for me to condense into a short description what it has meant to be a haemodialysis patient for the past 8 years, but I shall try to dwell on what, for me, have been the most important lessons and how my attitudes towards dialysis have changed and developed. I first became aware that all was not well when I was a preclinical medical student. My blood-pressure was found to be moderately raised during an experiment in a physiology practical. I was treated with 'Valium' and told that, being tall, I might need a slightly higher pressure anyway! Needless to say that wasn't the end of the story. A few months later I had an attack of acute glomerulo-nephritis and within 10 months was on a kidney machine. At first I was simply glad to be alive and appreciated the more liberal diet, but I could not honestly say that I felt much better. I was always tired and would often have episodes of hypotension. The diet was strict, unpalatable and seemingly inflexible. I have since learned, through my own experimentation, that there is much room for dietary manoeuvre and this has made an enormous difference to my quality of life. Since I was both a doctor and a patient, medical staff often had great difficulties in deciding on which level to deal with me. I was either told too little in a somewhat patronizing way, or not enough which left me confused and worried. I was often treated more as a set of biochemistry results than as a human being. Far too little attention was paid to my psychological needs which I was left to sort out for myself as best I could. The major drawbacks of dialysis are still tiredness, commitment to the machine, and the difficulties imposed by a diet.

After I qualified I started work in hospital but found that the rigours of being a houseman and coping with dialysis were too much. I became very tired and depressed and realized that I would have to search for some form of 'medical' work elsewhere.

Many dialysis patients look well but in a strange way this can be a disadvantage. One is competing as a 'normal' person whereas life on dialysis can never be normal and should not be considered so. The main worries that patients have are not so much about death or problems with vascular access, but more with the simple desire to be well and lead a normal life; haemodialysis has a very wearisome effect. I have always been totally independent about my dialysis, feeling that it is my responsibility and therefore up to me to carry it out successfully. However, I am still in my twenties and believe unquestioningly that transplantation offers the best hope of normal life and it is that desire which really keeps me going. I do not believe that a young person should be condemned to dialysis for any great length of time and consider that transplantation should always be vigorously pursued.

As a representative of the National Federation of Kidney Patients' Associations, my main concerns are about the small number of patients receiving treatment in the UK and the small number of kidney transplants that are performed. It is not a simple economic argument. Nephrologists are presumably deciding who will live and who will die, even though many claim that they are not turning patients away. What happens to patients who are either refused treatment or, more probably, never even referred for it? The answer is that they die quietly. The goals must be to ensure that all patients with kidney disease are referred for specialist assessment and that nobody eligible for treatment is turned away. Dialysis and transplantation, despite their disadvantages, are well proven and successful forms of treatment and patients should not be denied them on the basis of dubious selection criteria. Patients themselves must become more aware of their right to receive treatment, or at least to have a fair hearing.

Card campaigns to increase the supply of donor kidneys are part of the answer, but the real solution lies with the medical profession. Most usable kidneys end up in hospital incinerators because medical staff are simply not aware that they could be transplanted, or, if aware, they think that in some way the procedure for obtaining the organs is too complex and they do not have the desire or the courage to set the wheels in motion. The answer lies in education. The desperate need for kidney transplantation was never emphasized to me as a medical student and even the most up-to-date textbooks fail to mention it. Theoretically, if full use were made of all the available kidneys, we should have a diminishing dialysis population, not a growing one.

It is extremely important that medical students are better educated with stress being laid on the need for transplantation and for better dialysis facilities. This policy would take a little time to produce a result but could have the most miraculous effect on the treatment of end-stage renal disease in this country. Kidney patients, too, are uniting more than ever before to ensure that they get a better deal in the future. The position of the UK in the dialysis 'league' has slipped drastically and tragically over the past decade compared with the rest of Europe and the USA. I fear that the balance will not be redresssed quickly, but a determined effort must be made now – most importantly for the sake of the patients but also for the prestige and respectability of British medicine. Dialysis and transplantation are in an area of medicine where the UK lags behind the rest of the civilised world and the NHS and the medical profession is shamed by it.

18.4 CONTINUOUS AMBULATORY PERITONEAL DIALYSIS (CAPD)

I have been treated by continuous ambulatory peritoneal dialysis (CAPD) for about 18 months. The cause of my renal failure was glomerulonephritis which took 4 years from first symptoms of inflammation to run its course, despite steroid therapy. My previous health record was excellent, involving only normal childhood illnesses, and up to 4 months before renal failure developed I displayed few signs of ill health with only swollen ankles and occasional early morning vomiting. It was all the more of a shock therefore when I was informed of my impending kidney failure and that I would have to make preparations to accommodate dialysis. My layman's idea of the kidney patient was, I daresay, similar to the views held by the majority of the unaffected population, that such people were invalids kept in a limbo by machines and just able to stay alive until they could get a transplant. These views have been fostered over a long period by the media who always present kidney patients as objects of pity, perhaps with the best of fund raising motives in mind, but I was horrified to realize that I was to become one. I thought that my whole life would change and that machine dependency would end my working career. Although the possibility of renal failure had been an obvious end point for some time, I believe that, in common with most other patients, I had convinced myself that it wouldn't happen to me. The doubts and fears I had about the future were immeasurably compounded by reports in the newspapers at the time that kidney patients were dying because of shortages of machines and money. I realize now that these stories are perennial but I asked for, and got, reassurance and commitment from the London Hospital before I would believe that I had any future at all.

When I eventually entered hospital, my high blood urea concentration indicated rapid remedial action and a Tenckhoff catheter was inserted for peritoneal dialysis. CAPD was first mentioned to me by the consultant, who indicated to his houseman that I might be a suitable patient for the system but I was told that I could go onto either haemodialysis or CAPD. It was a very difficult decision indeed as I had little first hand knowledge of either method. I think the consultant sensed my dilemma because he stopped at the end of my bed on his way home one evening, without his white coat and entourage of housemen and students and spent half an hour explaining the facts to me and helping me to choose. I opted for CAPD as I valued the greater freedom it would give me and I loathed the idea of machine dependency. There was the added advantage that the Tenckhoff catheter was already in place. Having chosen, I was more or less committed to backing my own judgement and giving the system every opportunity to prove itself, accepting both its benefits and its disadvantages.

While still in hospital, one of the thoughts uppermost in my mind was that of employment. The more obvious side-effects of steroid therapy had already cost me a job with an international corporation which felt, perhaps correctly, that I was giving the wrong sort of company image to their customers during my extensive outside work. I was offered an effective demotion but resigned and remained unemployed for 6 months. The problem was that I could not pass employment medicals with protein-laden urine. Eventually, I secured a job as a sales manager but without life assurance or pension rights. At that time I had not developed renal failure and I assumed that a company would not allow a kidney patient to work for them in any kind of responsible job. In the event, my employer was very fair and was prepared to wait and see if I could handle my job on my return.

I found that adjusting to the demands made by CAPD was easy. Each change of fluid takes between 25 and 30 minutes, in my case four times a day. I wake half an hour earlier and go to sleep half an hour later than previously. One change is made at around 6 or 7 o'clock on my return home from work. The lunchtime change is a little more difficult. On days when I am working in the office, I use the toilets; if out of the office, which is more usual, I use a local hospital. The casualty sisters are invariably sympathetic and I have never once had any difficulty. On the contrary, on many occasions they have asked if they and one or two of their nursing colleagues can watch a fluid change as they have not seen CAPD before. My favourite hospital by the way, is one in the North Midlands where the nurses always insist you have a cup of tea after changing your bag!

Even within the four changes required daily, there is considerable flexibility. On odd occasions it is possible to miss a bag change completely without ill effect. Further, the lunchtime change can be missed and three changes made in the evening each with a time space of 2.5–3 hours giving the required total of four for the day. I would add that these are the exception rather than the rule, but they do demonstrate the measure of freedom that I have found within the system.

Here I come to the main advantage of the CAPD system which is, of course, the diet or lack of it. On my current regimen I am restricted to 80 g of protein, 80 mmol of sodium and 80 mmol of potassium per day. In reality, as long as I use common sense, I eat what I want. Over-indulgence in protein or sodium is quickly dialysed off providing the over-indulgence is not constant although I do keep a wary eye on high potassium foods and stay away mostly from chocolate and fruit juices. My fluid intake is not restricted and it was here that I discovered a strange side-effect of the CAPD system was, as the questioner put it, 'relentless'. He was comparing been changed during the previous three hours. I'm not sure yet whether this is an advantage or a disadvantage!

I was asked recently by a haemodialysis patient whether living with the CAPD system was, as the questioner put it, 'relentless'. He was comparing his system with mine, saying that when he had finished dialysing, he could forget all about it for a couple of days whereas mine went on and on with bag changes virtually every 5 hours. The changes actually become less obtrusive as time goes by and the CAPD routine fits into your life. It becomes an established part of a familiar pattern, almost like shaving each morning, sometimes slightly irksome but nothing that you would violently object to. In fact, the only time that problems do arise is when that routine is broken, for example when away from home on holiday. The same routine has to be followed but under very different circumstances. I have found that on a touring holiday, the time you can spend away from home is limited by the physical weight of the bags that are carried in the car with you. Ten days away means 80 kg of extra weight in the car and a lot of bulk, although it shrinks fairly rapidly as the bags are used. I prefer touring holidays as static ones tend to involve a lot of swimming and water sports in which, of course, CAPD patients cannot participate.

Whilst talking of the disadvantages of the system, the risk of peritonitis must rank as the most worrying. It must, however, be seen in perspective. The risk is ever present and must never be forgotten and taking even the smallest chance is not justified. But providing that the proper aseptic routine is followed and common sense precautions are observed the danger of infecting the system can be kept at bay. I have not suffered from peritonitis in the 18 months that I have used CAPD, and I attribute this to the good training received when I commenced on the system at the London Hospital together with a modicum of care since. As well as the aseptic routine, I talk to no-one when changing a bag, nor will I let anyone within 6 feet of me. I even hold my breath for as long as the plastic spike is exposed. Over-reaction perhaps but it appears to have worked. On several occasions in the past I have had the suspicion that I have had an infected system although this was not proved. On one occasion I thought that my shirt cuff had brushed against the spike, on another I found a tiny leak in one of the bags when it was refilling after use. In both cases I contacted the hospital immediately and they prescribed a course of antibiotic. A slide was also sent for clarification of possible infection. So as I say, the risk must never be taken for granted but should not be seen as so dangerous as to invalidate the system.

In trying to adjust my lifestyle to accommodate dialysis my wife was of inestimable help, but in being single-minded and positive it is easy to overlook the emotional stress caused to those around you. She developed headaches, sleeplessness and slight weight loss, all indications of worry and stress before I realized it was me who was causing it. As both she and I grew accustomed to CAPD the symptoms disappeared.

I resolved at the start to keep renal failure and the treatment I was on to myself because I regarded it as a personal thing and because the few close friends who knew acted with faint embarrassment towards me. I still try to maintain confidentiality to the point where very few of my workmates are aware of my condition and none of the customers I deal with are. This spares me from the overkindness of people who believe kidney patients must be wrapped in cotton wool and protected. In short, I can lead a reasonably normal life with a well controlled condition. I'm quite happy to do so until such time as the drugs used in the treatment of transplants improve. As a matter of fact, my employers paid me a great compliment in January this year. They enrolled me in the pension fund. They believe I'm going to make it to a long retirement, just like I do!

19

The ethics of tension
G. R. Dunstan

To place a discussion of ethics last in a symposium is to invite several wrong assumptions. One wrong assumption is that ethics does not matter. This would be wrong. Moral claims cannot be discerned until all the empirical features of a case are exposed. Another is that practitioners, the people we have heard for two days, read technical papers only, innocent of ethics. That would be wrong also. There are ethical judgements written into most of them, implicit if not always explicit.

A third might be that ethics is the same as politics, a matter of mobilizing forces to twist governmental arms. That would be too hasty. We need to reason our way through to an ethical conclusion before we pursue the politics.

The fourth assumption might be that ethics has to do with steering clear of the law; that ethical conduct is that which would give a doctor a good defence in court, and that unethical conduct is that which would cost him or his insurers heavy damages if not also a term in prison. That might be true in some countries. It is not yet true in the United Kingdom. Here we take ethics, medical ethics, to be more than medical etiquette, the conventions by which the profession regulates its own internal life, but it is not in itself a litigious exercise. It is the pursuit of equitable expectations between practitioners and patients, a pursuit in which a moderately informed lay public, including philosophers, the occasional theologian and socially interested lawyers, take their parts; but generally with the practitioners, not ranged against them. It is in this benign tradition of amicable joint pursuit that I stand here by invitation today; and I am grateful for the privilege.

Ethics for our purpose means moral judgement, coming to a right decision. For the practitioner, exercising professional judgement, the right

231

decision will generally be technical, an assessment of likely benefit and possible risk in the application of knowledge and skill to each patient's need. It may on occasion call for moral judgement also, when particular circumstances may raise the question whether the treatment specific to the ill is in fact the right treatment for this patient. For the patient an ethical stance may determine his consent and commitment to the treatment offered or his rejection of it. Much depends on the value he puts on his own life, or upon life of a given quality, as against other values which he holds. And for both practitioner and patient ethical judgement is very much shaped by social considerations: by the common morality, that is what the wider society holds to be right, or legal, or worthwhile, and is prepared to pay for.

To apply the word ethics to processes, therefore – to ask, for example, what is the ethics of continuous ambulatory peritoneal dialysis (CAPD)? – is to ask the wrong question. The ethics of CAPD is precisely that of any other therapy in a developmental stage, neither more nor less. The better question is, what factors have those moral agents involved in the treatment – practitioners, patients, administrators, allocators of funds – to reckon with in making right decisions? One factor common to them all is tension.

Considering the number of people expected to reduce it, tension must be reckoned on the whole to be a bad thing. We expect, against all experience, politicians and diplomatists to reduce international tension, policemen and community relations people to reduce social racial tension, doctors, soothsayers and priests to reduce personal tension. Yet life would be impossible without it, the moral life as well as the physical.

In ethics the really interesting questions arise not when good and bad, black and white, conflict, but when each of a cluster of good principles relevant to the matter in hand exerts its own claim. Moral reasoning is then required to resolve the tensions of these claims. The events in the Falkland Islands have given us a very good example outside the medical field: whether we should fight to regain the Falkland Islands or not. In the old just war tradition it is lawful to go to war *ad repetendas res* – to restore a position wrongfully overthrown. But there is also in the same tradition the principle that there must be a likelihood of success and the principle of proportion. If, in seeking to right the wrong, one will probably cause harm disproportionate to any good that might be attained, one must not do it. The ethical issues arising in the treatment of renal failure are, if I have heard aright, of this sort: the resolution of conflicting claims. They stand out most clearly from the papers touching the assessment of patients.

To the mind, the treatment of chronic renal failure is an intellectual whole, a notional progression through dialysis of one sort or another to renal transplant, repeated if required, though not every patient will go through the whole progression. Ideally selection of patients at any stage is a matter of clinical decision alone—to match each patient's unique condition with appropriate management. Diagnosticians are assumed to know which conditions, like diabetes, complicating the renal failure, indicate CAPD, now that it is available, in preference to haemodialysis. They are assumed to know which patients would do better still with a transplant and when the transition should be made. Information exists to tell them the relevance of the age factor, among others, at any stage. In fact, the ideal cannot always be realized. Clinical judgement has to compete for its validity with other claims, some personal to the patient and others the product of social policy.

I need do no more than mention the domestic and personal factors which may incline against selection for any particular form of dialysis. Some have been mentioned and some have been dismissed: unsuitable home, lack of domestic support, mental or physical impairment significant in a material respect, lack of dexterity with the catheter or lack of obsession with cleanliness so inviting peritonitis, and so on. These tell against selection simply as facts. To be Australia antigen positive is another adverse fact, but with a difference. The patient could be accepted for dialysis if, for the protection of other patients, the whole unit were duplicated in segregation on his behalf; and at once the resource factor comes in. But beyond these adverse facts there is another moral possibility. The patient is at liberty, in our general moral tradition, to decline the regime prescribed for him if it makes demands on his pattern of life which he is not prepared, for adequate reasons, to meet. He may judge the price of survival too high if it imposes social, dietary or other restrictions which he is unwilling to accept. This principle of autonomy – I said – is accepted, and therefore is to be respected, in the general moral tradition (Byrne, 1983). It was not so in the old Hippocratic tradition, in which the patient was expected to do as he was told (Polani, 1983). It is not so in the orthodox rabbinic Jewish ethical tradition which matches the Hippocratic, but for other reasons (Jacobovits, 1983). But it stands firm in the Catholic tradition of moral thinking (Soane, 1983) and in that dispersed convention of medical practice upheld in such declarations as those of the World Medical Association, Geneva 1948 and Helsinki 1975.

There is then a moral tension between what the doctor may properly prescribe and what the patient may as properly decline. Death is not for the patient the ultimate disaster nor for the doctor the ultimate failure. Recognition of this fact has practical value. A patient uncertain in his commitment to the regime is more likely to drop out and so to waste resources.

These contraindications, personal to the patient, must be annoying to the renal physician. But he is less frustrated by them, less provoked, than he is by the restraints of social policy and by the limitation of resources. Parsons and Lock (1980) in their survey of the grounds on which forty notional patients were rejected from a scatter of dialysis centres, argue, from the lack of clinical consistency in the rejections, that in fact diagnostic criteria are being used to translate economic and political decisions into rationing. Patients are rejected, they argue, not because they are unsuitable but because resources will not extend to treating them all. The same pressure is potentially at work if a patient is encouraged onwards, so to speak, from dialysis to transplant, primarily in order to make room for more dialysis patients.

This economic restraint is resented. Tension enters again, between the physician and the administrator, the provider of resources. Professor Oreo-poulos (see Chapter 6) erects the autonomy of the patient into an absolute. He says, 'Only the patient has the right to accept or reject a medical treat-ment'. To narrow the criteria for acceptance into treatment in order to ration treatment he says is immoral: it violates the whole tradition of medical ethics which he prays in aid. So, after urging saving, wherever savings can be made, and a concerted campaign to secure more finance for renal treatment, he would require a declaration from society and govern-ment as to 'whether or not expensive life-support systems should be pro-vided to everyone'. Here is tension indeed between the ideal, if upon reflection it is the ideal, and the real.

If we translate these words into another form, the government is hereby required to declare whether it puts upon the medical prolongation of every life a value, not absolute indeed, but higher than upon all or most of those other goods which government must provide. It is easy in contemporary rhetoric to contrast the provision for Trident nuclear weapons with pro-vision for whatever good cause the speaker has at heart: education, social services, the rebuilding of prisons, the unemployed. But rhetoric will not eliminate the tensions of a world which is not of the government's making. Granted that national defence is a duty of government, the cost of defence is what military technology now makes it, just as the cost of medicine is now what medical technology makes it; and it would be higher still if we turned back from the nuclear deterrent, whatever its merits or demerits, to reliance on conventional forces instead. And so government could argue, point by point, about each allocation of public expenditure, claim conflicting with claim. Without infinite gross national product or taxable wealth it cannot meet infinite claims. (I follow Dr Cattell (See Discussion Session 1) in directing pointed questions to the Confederation of British Industries and to the Trades Union Conference about increasing the national product if we want to increase the national benefit; but even so we will not reach infinity.) And if, within the health budget, the government met the claim for unrestricted treatment from the nephrologists, what answer is it to return to the cardiologists, the rheumatologists, the oncologists and the rest? When to do justice absolutely is impossible, we are driven to distributive justice, and so to selection, choice. And in the choice the calculation of risk, cost and benefit cannot be ruled out as sullying the professional mind. Effective cost analysis can in fact result in the saving of more lives (Mooney, 1980).

The renal surgeon has good cause too, as good as the physician, to resent the constraints of society. He is constrained in this country by the Human Tissue Act 1961, interpreted as liberally as it may be by the circulars of the DHSS. He depends for his supply of cadaver kidneys, matchable kidneys, on voluntary donation; and the donation rate falls every time lay and professional confidence in medical judgement is shaken by a tendentious television programme. It is not in dispute that he could obtain more kidneys and more quickly if he could take them from any suitable cadaver unless the deceased had contracted out, that is, expressly registered his refusal of consent before death. Why then is the law not changed to enact this common-sense solution? It is because of a justifiable fear of surrendering one more liberty to the authorities, whose tendency is, for administrative convenience, always to restrict liberty more and more. Between authority's will towards exaction and the subject's insistence upon his liberties – liberty for the sake of donation he would say at his best – there is inevitable tension.

The renal surgeon and his potential patient are at present the losers from that tension. It is not necessary to argue that the preservation of liberty must require that loss, for the libertarians have shown themselves rather weak in promoting donation by determined and effective means. Zeal for liberty might well engender more zeal for life. It is not uncommon in fact for the tension of conflicting claims to be broken by an ethical *démarche*, the insertion of a new thrust in positive action which breaks the deadlock of mutual contradiction. (A ready example of this is in the advance of clinical pharmacology in the control of pain, which rendered obsolete, for those who think about it, the old euthanasia debate and its conflict of claims – between the individual's interest in relief from prolonged pain and the common interest in restraining acts of killing or of suicide.) Tension, in short, is inescapable though assailable. Ethics consist, in part, in the equitable resolution of tension. The professional man cannot escape that duty; to seek to do so would be unethical.

Ethical issues have been thrown up in our discussions and I shall pick up two of them; indeed, I have been prodded to do so by the occasional conversation at table or on the terraces. First, Dr Frank Parsons (see Chapter 1) somewhat rhetorically set the cost of keeping convicted murderers in prison for life against the cost of prolonging the 'innocent' lives of renal patients. No man is on oath when he is speaking rhetorically, but if we were to take him seriously he would have us take some lives by judicial execution in order to spare others: that is, another form of selection to die. Thereby he would bring in a calculation of the entitlement to medical care; a criterion which we should not allow, as Professor Oreopoulos said, in any other medical decision. There is no escape from the tension of limited resources that way, if we are to adhere to our canon of medical treatment that a man is treated for his own self, irrespective of moral or social worth.

Secondly, Dr Ogg (see Chairman's Introduction, Session 2) quoted prosecuting counsel in the Arthur case to the effect that not to treat a treatable patient might constitute murder. (I am not a lawyer so my reflections must be received with caution. If I remind you that I am a moralist you may be even more cautious still. Ian Kennedy has written well on the subject and I am his debtor.) The Arthur case was not a strong one on which to ground any legal precedent. The Hammersmith case, *Re. B*, the baby Alexandra, decided in the Court of Appeal a few months earlier, in August 1981, was much stronger. And the words recalled, that not to treat a treatable patient might constitute murder, were words of the prosecuting counsel and not of the judge. Even so we may look at them.

The major ground of that prosecution, if I recall it correctly, was not simply the instruction to give nursing care only, but the administration of a drug in such quantities as to invite the inference of an intention to kill. In fact the jury declined to draw that inference and Dr Arthur was acquitted. But the point is worth recalling. The law distinguishes intent from motive. And intent is inferred from the material acts either admitted or proved: material *acts*, what is done. The question follows: could the omission of certain acts invite the same inference, of intent to kill? Or, less severely, could the omission be the ground of an action for negligence?

Now the duty required of a doctor is one of reasonable care, and reasonable care, reasonableness, is judged by what is recognized on the testimony of his professional peers to be appropriate management; management appropriate to that patient given the existing state of knowledge and the existing facilities. It is not appropriate management in all circumstances to seek to prolong life. There is no absolute right to life in our law and therefore no absolute duty to prolong it. Hippocrates said long ago that it was unphysicianly to attempt to treat the untreatable. For instance, in terminal care, or in the case of a very severely handicapped newlyborn child (and I do not include a Down's syndrome child in that description), invasive treatment is *not* held to be appropriate management. A doctor could be held negligent therefore only if he omitted to give treatment which he is already under a duty to give and can give. Where there is no such duty and no such possibility there is no negligence and no crime; or so I believe.

Now renal medicine is not to be equated with terminal care except in its final stages. A doctor, therefore, is still under duty to provide reasonable care appropriate to his patient. He has still to decide what is appropriate. But he need not, I believe, let the Arthur case add to his worries.

References

Byrne, P. A. (1983). Divergence on consent: a philosophical assay. In Dunstan, G. R. and Seller, M. J. (eds.). *Consent in Medicine: Convergence and Divergence in Tradition.* (In press) (London: King Edward's Hospital Fund)

Jacobovits, I. (1983). The doctor's duty to heal and the patient's consent in the Jewish tradition. In Dunstan, G. R. and Seller, M. J. (eds.). *Consent in Medicine: Convergence and Divergence in Tradition* (In press) (London: King Edward's Hospital Fund)

Mooney, G. H. (1980). Cost-benefit analysis and medical ethics. *J. Med. Ethics,* **6,** 177

Parsons, V. and Lock, P. (1980). Triage and the patient with renal failure. *J. Med. Ethics,* **6,** 173

Polani, P. E. (1983). The development of the concept and practice of patient consent. In Dunstan, G. R. and Seller, M. J. (eds.). *Consent in Medicine: Convergence and Divergence in Tradition* (In press) (London: King Edward's Hospital Fund)

Soane, B. (1983). Consent and practice in the Catholic tradition. In Dunstan, G. R. and Seller, M. J. (eds.). *Consent in Medicine: Convergence and Divergence in Tradition* (In press) (London: King Edward's Hospital Fund)

Discussion

H. Lupton (East Birmingham Hospital): Mr Page said that he was not able to swim. His CAPD nurses might be able to give him some advice about that. In Birmingham children have been swimming successfully with no complications.

R. Page: I am very pleased to hear it.

S. Taber (EDTNA): I have thoroughly enjoyed this multidisciplinary symposium. Over the last year there has been a fair amount of discussion about holding joint EDTA/EDTNA and European Dialysis Patients' Association Meetings. Can I ask what a member of the Patients' Association feels, what Dr Cattell feels and perhaps what Miss Winder feels about such joint meetings?

W. Cattell: Ms Taber is asking about the possibility of having a joint meeting of EDTA, which is primarily the professional group, EDTNA, which is the nurses, and a European patients' group.

Taber: There were actually a thousand patients in Paris and they formed themselves into an association.

B. Pearmain: Ms Taber is suggesting that the European patients should get organized to form a European association.

Taber: I thought that they had actually formed an association.

Pearmain: The German Patients' Association was the prime mover in starting a European patients' organization. It is still in the process of being organized and it is not a proper functioning body as far as we are concerned. It is difficult to describe why we are not particularly involved at the moment, but there are two national organizations that have been set up to represent patients. We understand that there is some doubt, or some confusion about which one should be involved, because there can only be one patients' association representing a national organization.

At the moment we are trying to sort out which should be our representative. We know which one rightfully represents the patients. Our problem at the moment is to persuade those that are setting up the European organization that what we say is the truth.

Cattell: I would like to address myself to the concept of a collective jamboree. I am perhaps the wrong person to ask as I have the reputation for calling a spade a bloody shovel.

Taber: That is why I asked.

Cattell: I can only give my personal opinion. Let me go, for those who do not know it, into the background history. The European Dialysis and Transplant Association was set up in Europe in 1964, and held its first meeting in Amsterdam. This was an association brought together to promote the development of dialysis and transplantation in Europe. Frank Parsons was one of its founder members. One of its major successes has been the development of the registry, which is quite unique.

As the years went by, nephrology was added. Frank Parsons may happily come in and correct me, but there has always been, to a greater or lesser extent, the suggestion by many of my colleagues in renal medicine that dialysis and transplantation is really for the non-scientific, the non-academic, not the true blue university type consultant, and nephrology was brought in to make it more honourable.

EDTNA followed and it was by this time apparent that the nurses, their artificial kidney assistants and many other people were in reality heavily involved in dialysis and that they could not be ignored. There were several misgivings about the creation of EDTNA because medicine is a very reactionary profession, and this was seen as a dilution of the integrity and the beauty of this European Association. It has, however, been shown to be successful. I certainly welcome these joint meetings and believe they are immensely important.

You are now taking it a step further. You are now asking should we also involve the patients? They are very articulate, they are very informed. As a population they are probably better informed about self-care, health care than anyone else.

Let me confess at this point that I am a considerable admirer of Ivan Illych (1975), and one of my roles in life is possibly to transfer health care away from hospitals and doctors to the patients themselves. Given this context, I believe that there is an evolving situation where we must in modern society involve the patients far more. I doubt, if one wants the hard reality, that any such proposal would be acceptable to more than 10 or 15% of my colleagues. But it is a jolly good idea.

Taber: May I consult Miss Winder on this aspect. In Paris we were told that it was a super idea but the hospital where they organized the nursing end of the meeting actually had on one day 14 extra patients to dialyse, and whereas they had thought they could send most of their staff to the meeting, they found that they were busy dialysing patients that had just turned up. This is why it may need to be properly thought out.

E. A. Winder: A three-way meeting of doctors, nurses and patients was not something that I had thought about. In a symposium, like this one, it works fantastically well, and we should encourage such meetings where we discuss attitudes from the patients' point of view. It is exceptionally good for nephrologists as well as nurses, although maybe the nurses hear what the patients have to say more on their own home ground. Listening to David Benoliel telling us how important it would have been to him to have had information about transplantation before he was transplanted is a tremendous lesson to all of us.

But I must admit that I am not sure that in a major once-a-year enormous meeting like EDTA/EDTNA, where we are really discussing slightly more scientific approaches, we should also be joined by a patient's association. It is a daunting proposition to think of organizing a meeting that large. I am not saying that it is impossible, but it would frighten me. But for meetings like this it is incredibly valuable.

Little: I certainly agree with Dr Cattell and I am glad he agrees with what I had to say about patient participation. Surely there are few other fields of medicine where patient participation is so important and so inevitable. More and more patients are educating themselves about dialysis. I would have thought that the obvious answer to the question about whether patients should participate is yes, inevitably.

D. Benoliel: My impression last year was that the meeting of patients was more like the Edinburgh Fringe. It happened around the EDTA/EDTNA meeting.

It would probably be a good idea but it should not be a big event. I think representatives from each country should attend and certainly participate in the nursing sessions and occasionally in the medical sessions. They should have their own small session with an invited speaker. I do not envisage that it would include a massive influx of patients from all over Europe.

The European associations did form an association in Paris last year but it is a bit like the EEC. We in Britain tend to be rather insular and other countries have very different problems from ours. We have a Health Service, which is a problem in itself but it also has certain benefits. Representatives from other countries were a little more militant in the things they were asking for. Perhaps we should be also. Discussions are continuing. I do not think the association will meet this year in Madrid, but perhaps the year after in London on our home ground. I think it would be a good idea.

A. M. Brownjohn (Leeds General Infirmary): What contribution do the patients' own family doctors or general practitioners make to their treatment at the moment, or is it totally managed by the hospital?

Page: Absolutely none. I cannot remember the last time I saw him.

Benoliel: My general practitioner was very flattered to be invited round to see my dialysis equipment and has been very helpful ever since. The problem is that he has rarely been sent up-to-date reports by the hospital. I think they sometimes take months and months to reach him. He rang me up about a year after my transplant to congratulate me because he had just been told. He is a very nice man and I get along with him very well.

It is understandable, I think, in a condition like renal disease that one needs very close medical contact with the renal unit and it is only natural that one should pick up the telephone every time one sneezes.

On that theme, I do feel that more use could be made of other people in the community team, like health visitors and district nurses. I do feel that they have a great role to play in visiting patients on their own territory and perhaps relieving some of the strain on the renal unit staff, caused by dialysis.

Pearmain: I cannot add any more to what has been said. My own GP fits into the already established pattern. If I get a problem that I can attribute directly to non-renal causes I go and see my GP. If I suspect it is renal – and one can only suspect because so many odd things turn up that are attributed to the renal problem generally – then I go to the unit.

I have been at home 8 years. There has been an open invitation to my GP to pop in any time he is passing to see the unit and have a rundown on how it works. He has not yet managed to find the time. Perhaps I have not given him long enough because I know GPs are busy. But I would have thought that perhaps he could have made it within 8 years.

The only other time that I have seen my GP in connection with a renal problem was one night when I was dialysing, and I was asleep, and I had a massive blood loss. The unit told me to get my GP in and the poor chap turned up. There was blood all over the place, my wife was trying to stay calm, I was out for the count anyway, and the poor guy tried to get some saline into me. At the end he was just looking at a mass of lines everywhere and asking my wife what goes in where. One could not help thinking afterwards that if he had come before to see it working rather than at 3 o'clock in the morning in an emergency he would have been able to take in the problem immediately and have done what was necessary. That was about 6 or 7 months after I had gone home. I was not then able to deal with that sort of problem very well, and neither was my wife.

I certainly would like to see GPs much more heavily involved. Perhaps patients' associations, local and national, can help to inform GPs and organize open days at renal units and symposia like this, say just for an afternoon. They can then be shown round the unit, and receive some sort of briefing about the likely problems that arise on home dialysis. It is an area where patients' associations could do a lot of good work.

Little: I agree with what Mr Pearmain says but there are limitations. GPs on the whole are notoriously ignorant about dialysis and about the treatment of renal failure in general. From my own point of view I have two problems. First, I am a doctor, so for minor problems I probably look after myself, and when it comes to nephrology then I know more about it than my GP – without wishing to sound arrogant. The answer is therefore no. I do not see my GP when it comes to medical problems, nephrological or otherwise.

Cattell: This is an area which has concerned a lot of us. It has been our practice, in theory and more or less in practice, over the last 15 to 16 years that every time we put a patient on regular dialysis we write to his family practitioner, inviting him to visit the unit, and inviting him to be involved with the day to day management of minor ills although we would accept total responsibility for the dialysis. In these 15 or 16 years we had a slight flurry of four or five GPs during the first 2 years. I certainly have not seen one in the last 5 years and I am very resentful.

I am not absolutely sure in my own mind – aside from a nice caring supportive family doctor attitude which patients need whether or not they are on dialysis – as to whether the family doctor has any significant role. Mr Pearmain feels that he should be involved. What about the other two?

Page: To me, particularly on CAPD, no. The sort of problems that crop up with CAPD could only be handled by the unit.

Benoliel: No, I thought I had made it reasonably clear. I do not think the GP should be involved in medical matters concerning dialysis because these are normally rather immediate and need to be dealt with by the hospital, and what may not appear related to the renal condition very often is. The medical treatment should come from the hospital, but I still support what I said about community nursing and health visiting support.

Winder: I should like to comment on the involvement of community or district nurses, which I think a lot of units have tried in several different ways. I would be inclined to agree with Dr Cattell about GP input. It is a very nice idea for community or district nurses to be involved to the extent of knowing if they have dialysis patients on their patch and making visits in order to see that they are happy and well. But I would be very anxious about district or community nurses getting involved in any aspect of the actual technicalities of dialysis. The trouble is that if they are involved in a social respect they tend to want to get involved and the patients tend to want to use them.

It interested and amused me that Dr Little said that the only time his fistula had ever been blown was when a nurse needled it. That does not surprise me at all. He should be better at it than the nurse. What worries me is when a patient on home dialysis who lives a long way away from a unit needs to have help with his needling and then calls the district nurse or community nurse who happens to have made contact. We have had problems in our unit and I have heard horrendous stories of the awful things that have happened when both GPs and district nurses or health visitors have got involved in something that they do not understand.

A London hospital home dialysis patient went to his GP with an infected fistula and the GP lanced the boil!

C. Wight: (Addenbrooke's Hospital): Before I became a transplant co-ordinator I was a health visitor. I went to college for a year and I learnt about health visiting after a full nursing training. There were several patients within the practice for which I was working who were on dialysis or who had had a transplant and we had never been told. I felt cheated as a health visitor. These were people who had come to a new illness, a crisis that we heard the social worker talking about earlier, and I think a health visitor could have been very helpful at home. Certainly the general practitioners never told their health visitor that these people existed, and it was part of my duty in the community to follow up people who needed help.

J. Auer: As hospital social worker at the Churchill I do liaise quite a lot with health visitors, especially with the group of patients who have multiple medical problems such as the diabetics or the paraplegics who require dressings. It is not a common policy to inform health visitors as a routine, but they should be informed for the very reasons that have been mentioned. So often there are problems with children in the family at the same time and the health visitor ought to be aware of all patients on dialysis, including CAPD and transplant patients.

I have one further point about GPs. There have been several references to late referrals from GPs over the past 2 days. There have been references also to the need for preventive work which would presumably start at the primary health care level. I would have thought that if this bad blood between the GPs and the renal units continues, then I can see no possibility of a GP referring a patient early in the course of renal disease. How are they likely to know? How can they refer? And how can they be involved in preventive work if there is bad blood between GPs and renal units?

Cattell: I almost thought of handing this problem to Professor Dunstan to sort out the bad blood or the tensions between hospital doctors and family doctors. I am not sure that this is a feature peculiar to dialysis. It may heighten it. One of the sad things is that there is this separation throughout health care between hospital doctors and non-hospital doctors.

R. Dowie (St Leonard's Hospital): I should like to comment on general practitioners' attitudes to chronic renal failure. I have interviewed 45 general practitioners recently. I was particularly interested in the whole concept of their relationships with consultants across all specialties and the referral process. What came out quite clearly was their general lack of awareness of the potential for nephrologists to provide successful treatment to patients who have reached end-stage. I asked them to keep a record of all referrals made in the week prior to my seeing them, and whilst I had numerous referrals recounted to me of urinary complaints that had been referred to urologists, only one referral had gone to the renal physicians. And what was evident in their comments was a general belief that end-stage renal failure is terminal, and in a short-term sense. I will not say it is universal, but certainly there were elliptical comments to the point that they felt that if a patient reached that particular department the long-term future was not good.

It seems that we really are going back to the point that Dr Little was making, about training general practitioners or, indeed, the whole of the medical profession whilst they are still students. It is not just a question of general practitioners referring patients late. I think they are also being referred late to nephrology departments from other specialties within the hospital, within an individual hospital and between hospitals. I do not think it is quite fair to hit the GP quite so hard when we are perhaps looking at intra-professional ignorance.

F. M. Parsons (Leeds General Infirmary): I did a calculation for Leeds which has 200 GPs and it worked out that a GP would see about one new patient on his panel with end-stage renal failure in 10 years. That is the average incidence of renal disease in general practice. I do not think it is very practical to train GPs in dialysis technology which alters continuously as time goes by.

Home dialysis frequently takes place in the evening or overnight. If patients in Leeds ring GPs at this time they will get the emergency service. I leave what will happen to the imagination.

Cattell: We have had enough scary stories!

H. Lupton (East Birmingham Hospital): I have one GP who has three dialysis patients. By chance he was lucky enough to work in a renal unit before he became a GP, therefore his level of interest is obviously much higher than average. But he is interested. We have good telephone communication. And I find it marvellous to have a GP who has some knowledge and some interest in his patients.

I would love to communicate better with my GPs. I do not think they need 'training' in dialysis. All they need is an explanation of the basic principle – the blood comes out here along these lines through the dialyser and back in.

I have another GP who occasionally helps a patient out with needling. I have another GP who phoned me because a patient turned up on his doorstep with a blue toe and he did not know what to do with it. I am quite happy to give telephone information and advice. I think it is wonderful to have GPs involved. I would be very glad to see any GP coming to have a look at the unit and I think that patients should invite their GPs to come and have a look, perhaps even drag them to the unit.

Cattell: That is a nice note to end on. Be kind to your GP!

DR CATTELL'S CLOSING REMARKS

Before we go, it has occurred to me, although I have had no brief in respect of this, that it would be discourteous of us if we did not acknowledge Travenol Laboratories for setting up this symposium. They have a long and very honourable association with dialysis. Yes, they market a good piece of goods which I use. My experience has been that they are a most exemplary firm working in this area.

I should like to make special mention of Jeannette Robertson-Lomax and Alan Barrell both of whom I have found immensely helpful, and I am sure they have worked extremely hard on our behalf.

References

Gordon, P. M. and Cattell, W. R. (1970). Home conditions – the limiting factor in domiciliary dialysis. *Proc. Eur. Dial. Transplant Assoc.*, 7, 248
Illych, I. (1975). *Medical Nemesis.* (London: Calder and Boyars)

Index